By the Editors of Consumer Guide®

MEDICAL BOOK OF REMEDIES:

50 Ways to
COPE WITH
ARTHRITIS

Written by
DIANA L. ANDERSON, R.N., M.S.N.

Consultant: Paul Katz, M.D.
Georgetown University Medical Center

PUBLICATIONS INTERNATIONAL, LTD.

Louis Weber, C.E.O
Publications International, Ltd.
7373 North Cicero Avenue
Lincolnwood, Illinois 60646

Permission is never granted for commercial purposes.

Manufactured in U.S.A.

8 7 6 5 4 3 2 1

ISBN: 0-7853-1172-6

Contributors:

Diana L. Anderson is first vice president of the Association of Rheumatology Health Professionals, director of the outpatient Bone and Joint Center at St. Paul Medical Center, and chief operating officer of Metroplex Clinical Research Center in Dallas, Texas.

Paul Katz, M.D., (consultant) is professor and vice chairman of the Department of Medicine and chief of the Division of Rheumatology, Immunology, and Allergy at Georgetown University Medical Center. Dr. Katz serves on the Council on Education of the American College of Rheumatology and is a member of the Government Affairs Committee of the Arthritis Foundation.

Illustrator: David Scanlan

CONTENTS

CONTENTS

INTRODUCTION

You can do more than simply live with arthritis. You can live *well* with arthritis. Although the cause of and cure for most forms of arthritis are unknown, remarkable progress has been made in controlling the effects of these diseases. And you can take advantage of that progress. You can also take advantage of many of the techniques that health experts and people with arthritis have developed through the years to cope with the disease.

First, of course, you need to get a diagnosis from a specialist and follow the doctor's recommendations and prescriptions. With prompt treatment, arthritis can usually be brought under control before it causes disability.

Also essential to living well with arthritis, however, is the depth of your involvement in your own care. That's where this book comes in. *50 Ways to Cope with Arthritis* gives you expert advice to help you participate more effectively in your own care. You'll find practical self-help tips for easing pain and stiffness. You'll find instructions for safe exercises, which are essential for maintaining function in arthritic joints. To help you fight fatigue and prevent unnecessary wear and tear on your joints, we give concrete suggestions for making your days "joint friendly." You'll learn how to plan and organize so you can conserve energy and how to make activities such as cooking, cleaning, and writing easier on your joints. You'll also find advice on dealing with the emotional aspects of coping with arthritis, making smart dietary choices that give your body the best chance at working well, and taking advantage of resources that can make living with arthritis easier.

We encourage you to read the entire book first, so you get an overview of the many aspects of arthritis self-care. Then go back and choose the remedies that are most appropriate for you. Remember to discuss your plans for change with your doctor first. Then go ahead and start taking back control of your life.

1 KNOW WHAT TYPE YOU HAVE.

For most people, the word "arthritis" conjures up an image of a gray-haired individual clutching painful, misshapen knuckles. While some people with arthritis fit this picture, many do not.

There are actually more than 100 types of arthritis. And while some forms primarily appear in the later years, some strike younger adults and children. The two most common forms are osteoarthritis and rheumatoid arthritis. These two forms will be the focus in this book (although many of the remedies may be applicable to other forms of arthritis). Knowing which type you have and what you might expect from it can help you do a better job of coping and maintaining greater control. While you'll need a diagnosis from a qualified physician (see remedy 2), the following information will give you an overview of your disease.

Let's start with osteoarthritis (OA), since it is most common. If you were to look at joint X rays of everyone over age 65, most of them would show some joint changes associated with OA, although many of those people would not have any symptoms. About 11 percent of the general population over age 65 show more severe joint changes that *are* accompanied by OA symptoms.

OA occurs as a result of a wearing down of the cartilage in the joints over time. In a normal joint, the ends of the bones are covered with cartilage, a durable, elastic tissue that protects the bones and allows the joint to move freely. Cartilage gets the oxygen and nutrients it needs by absorbing them, like a sponge, from the joint fluid. As the joint bends, waste products are squeezed out of the cartilage; as the joint relaxes, nutrients and oxygen are absorbed. (Controlled movement, therefore, benefits the joints.)

NORMAL JOINT ANATOMY

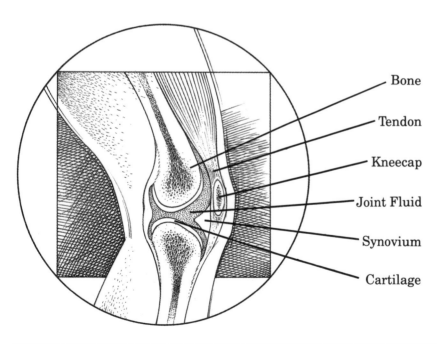

Bone

Tendon

Kneecap

Joint Fluid

Synovium

Cartilage

In OA, the cartilage thins out and may even wear away, leaving areas where bones rub directly against each other. The edges of the bones may thicken and form bony swellings known as osteophytes. Stiffness and dull pain in the joints with little or no inflammation are generally the result. These are the typical symptoms of OA.

The weight-bearing joints (hips, knees, and spine) are most frequently involved in OA. Other joints often affected are the finger joints closest to the tips of the fingers, which may develop bony knobs. The joint at the base of the thumb and the big-toe joint may also be affected. Osteoarthritis rarely affects the wrists, elbows, shoulders, ankles, or jaw. While OA may affect more than one joint at a time, the disease does not affect other systems or organs of the body.

OA is a chronic disease, but it may not necessarily get progressively worse, and many people with OA are relatively free of symptoms. Few people are severely disabled by the disease. Treatment for OA generally involves prescribed exercises to help keep the joints flexible and strengthen surrounding tissues, joint protection, and when necessary, medication and nondrug therapies to ease discomfort.

In contrast to OA, the hallmark of rheumatoid arthritis (RA) is inflammation. In RA, the lining of the joints, called the synovium, becomes inflamed. The synovium normally produces a fluid that lubricates the joint.

While the cause of RA is unknown, it is thought that the symptoms are the result of the body turning against itself. The immune system normally protects the body from invaders. In RA, immune-system cells are thought to be responsible for the inflammation. This is referred to as an autoimmune reaction.

The symptoms and course of RA vary from person to person. In its mildest form, it causes only minor joint discomfort and does not lead to serious joint impairment. More often, however, the inflammation causes painful, stiff, swollen joints. Prolonged inflammation of the synovium can lead to actual and sometimes severe joint damage. It can also destroy cartilage within the joint, weaken nearby ligaments and tendons, and cause painful spasms in muscles in the area. And, unlike OA, RA tends to affect other organs and systems, in addition to the joints. It can cause "body-wide" symptoms such as fatigue, fever, and weight loss. In its most severe form, RA can damage the heart, lungs, skin, blood vessels, nerves, and eyes.

RA usually develops between the ages of 20 and 50, although one form affects children and young adults. It is more common in women than in men. RA is usually chronic, although current treatment methods can sometimes put the disease in remission and can usually relieve pain and prevent deformities far better than treatment used a few years ago.

Most people with RA require medications. Drugs used include aspirin and similar anti-inflammatories, drugs that affect the immune system (gold salts, penicillamine, antimalarials, and methotrexate, for example), and, when necessary, steroids. In some cases, surgery may be done to correct joint deformities and relieve severe pain. As with OA, prescribed exercise and joint protection are essential aspects of treatment. Most people with RA do well and lead fairly normal lives.

CONSULT A PRO.

2

If you suspect you have arthritis but have not been diagnosed, get yourself to a qualified doctor. Many of us experience aches and pains associated with overuse of muscles and joints, illness, and the like. However, when aches and pains persist beyond a few weeks or when pain or stiffness is severe enough to interfere with everyday tasks, it's time to seek medical attention.

You don't have to learn to "live with" pain, nor should you just accept arthritis as a fact of aging without taking steps to protect your joints from further damage. Indeed, pain is the most common symptom that brings people to seek help for their arthritis. Unfortunately, the average length of time between onset of symptoms and medical intervention is four years. By that time, damage to the joints may have already occurred. So why not be "above average" and take your symptoms to a pro now.

Whom you take your symptoms to is also important. Some forms of rheumatic disease are difficult to diagnose, especially during the early stages of the disease process. So while your family physician may be your first contact, you may also require the expertise of a rheumatologist. A rheumatologist is an internist or pediatrician who has taken additional training in the area of arthritis and related disorders of the joints, muscles, and bones. Rheumatologists have devoted an additional two to three years of training after medical school to the study and care of rheumatic diseases. As a consultant, the rheumatologist will communicate directly with your family doctor in the management of your arthritis.

Your family doctor may refer you to a board-certified rheumatologist. You may also be able to get information about rheumatologists in your area from your local Arthritis Foundation (see remedy 45). Be sure the rheumatologist you choose is one whom you feel comfortable with and who is willing to thoroughly discuss your condition and its treatment with you.

Whether your condition is simple or complicated, early diagnosis and treatment is still the key to control and long-term management of your arthritis. And no matter how diligent you are at following the self-care tips in this book, your physician's expertise and advice is invaluable.

3 | BE A TEAM PLAYER.

In some cases, the best way to manage arthritis is to assemble a team of health-care professionals. As discussed in remedy 2, your family physician may refer you to a rheumatologist for evaluation, and together they will help you establish a treatment plan. The rheumatologist, in turn, may suggest that you work with other trained professionals, such as a physical therapist, occupational therapist, nurse, and social worker. Each team member has a responsibility and a role to play in helping people with arthritis lead the most productive lives possible. You may want to talk with your doctors about whether the following individuals could help you manage your arthritis:

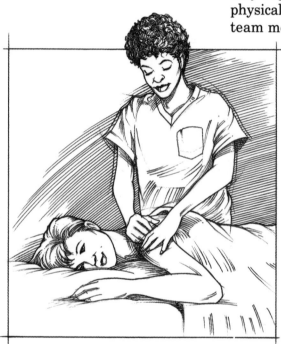

- **Physical therapist (PT).** The role of the PT includes helping to relieve pain and stiffness, suppress inflammation, prevent deformity, and maintain function through the use of nondrug therapies such as heat and ice treatments, massage, electrostimulation, and controlled movement of joints. The PT can also work with you to design an exercise program suited to your specific needs and interests (see remedies 17–24). The PT may also recommend the use of equipment, such as weights, pulleys, or traction, to assist you.

- **Occupational therapist (OT).** The OT is trained to do evaluations to determine which joints are affected by arthritis, to teach you ways to protect your joints from stress, and to help determine how much improvement you can expect. One role of the OT is to help people with arthritis to perform their daily activities more comfortably. The OT can offer suggestions on making everything from getting out of bed to getting dressed easier. Maybe you have trouble bathing, getting out of a chair, or putting on your shoes and socks, for instance; an OT can help you learn to use assistive devices and other forms of support to better accomplish these everyday tasks.

- **Nurse.** You will probably interact with the nurse in your doctor's office. The nurse should serve as your link to the doctor when you are away from the doctor's office and a question arises about your condition or its treatment. Oftentimes, when patients call the office, it is the office nurse who assesses the urgency of their need for an appointment. The nurse may also be involved in patient education. In addition, the nurse can provide psychological support and reassurance, physical evaluation and assessment, medication administration, and appraisal of needs in the home. In many instances, the nurse plays an important role in coordinating the services a patient may need. The role of the nurse may vary greatly depending on the setting. In some situations, a nurse practitioner may actually be the manager of the patient's condition.

- **Social worker.** The skills of the social worker are used in two main ways in the management of arthritis. Social workers provide counseling and support regarding social and emotional issues related to chronic disease. They are also trained to coordinate and facilitate access to community resources to meet emotional, physical, and financial needs. These professionals are also knowledgeable about insurance, disability, Medicare, and financial aid.

In addition to these health professionals, you must not underestimate your own role in the ongoing care of your arthritis. In actuality, *you* are the most important member of your health-care team. The primary goal of the team should be educating you and your family to be active participants in achieving and maintaining the highest level of independence possible.

Most people need to begin their plan to be healthier with additional education about their specific health problems and needs. As a patient, you are not required to have the same level of understanding about your disease as your health-care providers do, but studies have shown that well-educated patients are more likely to take proper care of themselves and therefore obtain the maximum benefit from treatment. So read on, and start taking a more active role in the care of your arthritis today!

4

PACE YOURSELF.

FYI

One way to help stave off fatigue is to learn how to conserve energy in your daily activities. You'll find helpful tips to do just that in remedies 25–35.

Coping with the persistent pain of arthritis—and dealing with the ups and downs of a chronic and often unpredictable disease—can be exhausting. Fatigue, in turn, can decrease tolerance to pain. That's why, for the person with arthritis, getting adequate rest is just as important as getting enough appropriate exercise. Achieving a balance between rest and activity is called pacing.

Some experts feel that the person with arthritis needs from 10 to 12 hours of rest per day. Some further suggest that this be broken down into eight hours of sleep at night and two 1-hour rest periods during the day. The need for rest, however, is a highly individualized matter. And it is important for you to determine—and respect—the amount of rest you need. If you're used to an active, busy life, it can be difficult to respond to that need for additional rest. But it's important to remember that forcing yourself to rest *before* you are exhausted can improve your endurance and comfort level over the long haul.

Resting does not necessarily mean sleeping. It means getting yourself as comfortable as possible, with your joints well supported in their normal position. Some people with arthritis wear specially made splints during rest periods to keep their joints in proper position.

Here are some tips to help you pace yourself:

- Schedule rest periods. You make appointments for work or to take your pet to the vet. Do the same for rest periods. It may help, at first, to schedule your day on paper, with rest periods marked in.

- Make it a habit. Rest is as essential as eating.

- Learn to say no, or at least to modify. Make things easy on yourself if you are going through a period of stress or pain. Go to that potluck, but take something easy to prepare. If you are planning a fatiguing activity, get plenty of rest before and after.

- If obligations make it difficult to spend an hour resting, take several shorter breaks throughout the day.

USE ICE TO REDUCE PAIN AND INFLAMMATION.

5

Although heat is used more widely, some people get relief from arthritis pain through the numbing effects of cold. Cold produces a sensation of numbness and has been used effectively to reduce both pain and muscle spasm in arthritis.

Although the first few minutes of cold treatment can be a bit uncomfortable, if you can make it through them, you may be surprised at the pain relief you achieve. As a guide, try applying the ice until numbness occurs. However, if the initial discomfort persists and the ice treatment feels like sheer torture, discontinue the treatment.

There are a variety of ways to apply cold treatment, including ice packs made by filling resealable plastic bags with ice, cold soaks, commercial ice products, and ethyl chloride spray. You can even make a handy reusable ice pack out of a bag of frozen vegetables, such as peas. When using an ice pack, you may find it more comfortable to wrap the pack in a thin towel before applying it to the joint.

Another technique for applying cold treatment is ice massage. This is an easy, economical way to apply ice to your joints. To make the ice massager, simply fill a Styrofoam cup with water and freeze. When you are ready to use it, peel the lip from the cup. This way, you have a flat surface of ice to apply to the joint and you have a holder that will keep your fingers from freezing as you apply the treatment. Apply the ice directly to the joints for five to seven minutes to help relieve pain.

Yet another option for relief from pain and swelling is the contrast bath. With this technique, you alternate hot and cold treatments. This can be done by alternating cold packs with a heating pad or, especially for the extremities, by placing the affected joint under running water, alternating the temperature of the water between hot and cold (if you use running water, however, be sure your water heater is set low enough to prevent scalding).

6 TRY HEAT.

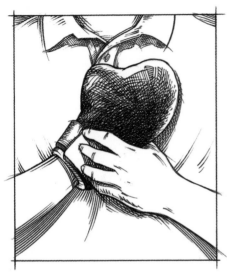

Heat treatment, especially moist heat, can also soothe arthritis pain and reduce or prevent stiffness. Because it helps to relax and loosen joints, heat can be especially beneficial before exercising or when you are trying to fall asleep.

A hot bath or shower or a dip in a warm pool or Jacuzzi are common ways to apply moist heat to the joints. You can also make hot packs using towels that have been soaked in hot water. Heating pads can be effective, but damp heat usually gives more relief. Commercial hot packs can also be purchased at pharmacies. Most of these are inexpensive, easy to use, reusable, and portable.

To prevent stiffness, it's also important to protect your joints from cold (unless you're applying cold treatment to ease pain). If you'll be in an environment where you cannot control the temperature, be prepared by carrying a sweater or jacket, spare socks, or even a pair of gloves. You might even try warming mitts, like those used by hunters and skiers, to keep your finger joints warm.

7 BE PREPARED FOR NIGHT PAIN.

FYI

A little TLC from a family member may help soothe and relax you enough for sleep. Ask for a back or neck massage or even just a gentle embrace.

These strategies may help you cope with nighttime arthritis pain:

- Take a warm bath or shower prior to sleep.

- Play soft music to distract you and induce sleep.

- Wait until you feel sleepy to hit the sack.

- Take your pain medication as directed. Talk to your doctor about scheduling a nighttime dose to help you sleep.

- Be sure you have a comfortable, supportive mattress and pillow, and make sure you're warm enough. Consider using an electric blanket.

MOVE TO PREVENT PAIN.

8

If you've read remedy 1, you know that moving the joints is the only way to nourish and lubricate them. Although keeping an arthritic joint in a stationary position may temporarily prevent pain, this extended lack of movement can produce greater pain and stiffness in the long run. In severe cases of lack of joint movement, contractures may develop. Contractures refer to shortening of the muscles and shrinking of the connective tissue. Over time, the joint's ability to function is reduced.

Gentle range-of-motion exercise as well as other types of more vigorous exercise (discussed in remedies 17–24) can help nourish the joints and prevent stiffness and pain. These should be performed regularly. In addition, try the following:

- Stretch frequently. Even during rest breaks, gently flex or stretch your joints occasionally or change your position slightly to prevent stiffness.

- Massage your joints. Massage can help soothe a painful area, and you'll be moving other joints as you do so (see remedy 12).

- If you'll be travelling by airplane, bus, or train or if you'll be sitting at a sporting event, concert, or movie, try to get an aisle seat. This will give you more room to stretch your legs frequently while seated. It will also make it easier for you to get up and move around once in a while.

- During long car trips, take advantage of rest stops to stretch and move around. If you're the passenger, do range-of-motion exercises for your fingers, lower legs, and neck while on the road.

- Avoid clenching objects for extended periods. If holding a pen is painful, try a computer or typewriter. Instead of holding a newspaper or book in your hands while reading, try laying it flat on a table or using a book stand. Instead of carrying a purse or briefcase with a handle, choose one with a shoulder strap.

9 PAMPER PAIN-PRONE FEET.

If you have arthritis in your feet, you know there is almost nothing worse than this type of pain. And since walking is pretty much required of all of us, it's essential to find ways to "out step" this foot discomfort.

Although some foot problems eventually require surgery, many surgeons recommend that you "shoe around" your bone spurs, bunions, and painful joint problems as long as possible. Surgery on the feet is often painful, tends to have a long recovery period, and does not have guaranteed results. Therefore, one of the most important steps you can take to prevent or decrease foot pain is to wear comfortable shoes.

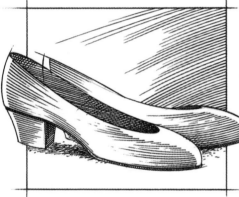

If you're a woman who would like to continue to wear a shoe with a heel, you may be able to do so as long as you choose wisely. Skip the pointy-toed, spike-heeled variety that provide little support even for normal feet, and opt instead for a lower, thicker heel that provides better stability. For special "high-heeled" occasions, bring along a lower-heeled pair to slip on after the event. You might even consider the newly available shoes with removable heels in low, medium, and high. This type of shoe allows you to change your heel height in the middle of an evening.

There are more comfortable options for men as well. Several companies now make dress shoes that look classy but are less binding. Some feature more flexible soles and uppers and more cushioning.

When shopping for shoes, look for:

- Heels that are no more than an inch in height for everyday wear. Chunkier heels are preferable to thinner ones.

- A wide toe area that does not put pressure on the toes.

- Shoes with uppers made of soft materials that will stretch somewhat to reduce pressure and accommodate swelling.

- Shoes that have laces or Velcro closures that can be loosened if your feet swell.

- An upper made of breathable material such as leather or canvas to help prevent foot ulcers, which may lead to infection.

Consider wearing athletic shoes whenever possible. These generally provide good support for the foot and ankle and have wide toe boxes and plenty of cushioning.

Another option in the prevention of foot pain is to have a podiatrist or orthotist design supports for your shoes. Arthritis of the foot often causes painful pressure points on or around the sharp edges of the bones, particularly if suitable shoes are not being worn. Orthotics can be designed to help prevent pressure points and provide support. Newer orthotics are lightweight yet durable and still provide needed stability. You can also find a variety of soft cushion inserts and corn and bunion pads at drug stores to help make your footwear more comfortable.

Sometimes, specially designed shoes are necessary, particularly for the person with rheumatoid arthritis. These shoes may be expensive, but depending on your insurance coverage, they may be reimbursable. An investment in a comfortable shoe with the proper support may be well worth the increased mobility and decreased pain.

In addition to choosing footwear carefully, there are also some techniques you can use to soothe and pamper your feet.

- Try nourishing the joints in your feet and ankles several times a day with the following routine. Flex your foot upwards and downwards from the ankles, scrunch your toes under and then point them, trace circles in the air with your toes, then spread your toes as far apart as possible and bring them together again.

- When you get home in the evening, try this exercise to relax your feet. Sit down and spread a dish towel on the floor in front of you. Put your heel down on the closest edge of the towel. Keeping the heel on the floor, pull the rest of the towel under your foot by scrunching your toes and arching your foot.

- When your feet are tired, give them a massage or, better yet, ask your partner to massage them for you. Use circular motions with your fingers to massage the tops and bottoms of your feet.

- Soak achy feet in a tub of warm water or in a commercial foot bath that has a massaging feature.

10   LEARN ABOUT THE RELATIONSHIP BETWEEN STRESS AND PAIN.

When we think of stress, we usually think of the negative kind, such as that associated with losing a job or having marital difficulties. But positive, pleasant events, such as a promotion or the birth of a child, can be equally taxing. These types of stress are a normal part of all of our lives. A chronic disease such as arthritis, however, can add a whole new set of stressors that, if not recognized and dealt with, can further aggravate the disease.

The person with arthritis often must deal with persistent pain, changing body image, some loss of function or mobility, and perhaps loss of self-esteem. These stressors can wear away at the body, causing fatigue as well as increased sensitivity and lower tolerance to pain. In essence, the person with arthritis can get caught in a pain-stress-pain cycle.

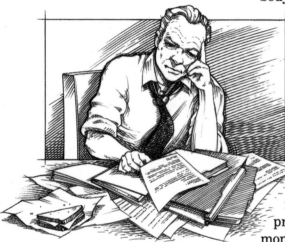

The perception of stress is highly individual. For someone who tends to be more laid back, a day at the beach can be relaxing and stress relieving. For someone who enjoys and thrives on excitement and who prefers to keep busy all the time, "taking it easy" at the beach may feel frustrating, nonproductive, and upsetting.

Still, when we experience something as stressful, whether it is physically or emotionally stressful, the body responds internally in some predictable ways. This response includes the release of the stress hormones adrenaline and cortisone. These hormones travel through the body, causing a variety of physical effects, such as increased heart rate and muscle tension. Researchers believe that when these reactions are ongoing—in other words, when stress is persistent—they take a physical toll. Research has shown that stress affects the immune system, which may increase our vulnerability to disease. And both emotional and physical stress appear to be able to trigger flare-ups of rheumatoid arthritis. In addition, the tension and fatigue that result from stress can play a large role in how pain is experienced, increasing sensitivity and creating even more stress.

Learning to recognize and cope with potential sources of stress in daily life may help break the pain-stress-pain cycle and help keep stress from further aggravating arthritis symptoms. Just as sources of stress vary somewhat for each person, so do the signs and symptoms of unregulated stress. The symptoms may be physical, such as a muscle spasm in the neck, tightness in the shoulders, upset stomach, skin rashes, rapid heartbeat and increased sweating, or difficulty breathing. They can also be emotional, such as irritability, outbursts of anger, depression, and anxiety. Sometimes, behavioral changes, such as increased alcohol consumption, overeating or loss of desire to eat, increased smoking, drug use, or decrease in sex drive can be signs of an overload of stress. Because the signs and symptoms of stress can vary so much, you need to be alert to the possibility that that pain in your neck, that blue mood you've been in, or the fact that you've hit the ice cream parlor every day this week may be a sign that you're under too much stress and that you need to take steps to try and cope with it.

Once you've recognized that you're stressed, you need to initiate some healthful strategies to decrease stress as much as possible or cope with it if you can't decrease it. Some suggested strategies that will be discussed in this book include exercising; participating in recreational activities; using relaxation techniques such as deep breathing, guided imagery, or biofeedback; having a massage; taking advantage of a support system (whether for an ear to listen or for a helping hand to relieve some burdens); learning to set priorities and to say no; and anticipating and preparing yourself for unavoidable stressful situations. You will need to tailor your coping methods to your needs and preferences, perhaps using several techniques to keep a reign on stress. The key, of course, is to recognize when it's time to put these strategies in action. If you can identify and work toward dissipating stress, you will have greater control over your arthritis.

TRY BREAKING THE PAIN-STRESS CYCLE WITH RELAXATION TECHNIQUES.

If you've read remedy 10, you know that stress can affect your arthritis and increase your discomfort. To help you manage stress and relieve the resulting tension and pain, you may want to try one of several relaxation methods. Keep in mind that no single relaxation technique works for everyone, so if you try one of these methods and feel uncomfortable with it, give another one a shot. If none of them seems to fit your needs, you may find that engaging in exercise or a hobby or just taking a few moments to sit quietly will work. Sometimes it is helpful to teach a friend or relative about your relaxation technique so they can help guide you or remind you to use the technique during stressful times or painful flares.

Although relaxation techniques are useful when you start noticing signs of stress, practicing relaxation as part of your daily routine can help to keep stress from building to an uncomfortable level and may even increase your tolerance to arthritis pain. Relaxation techniques can be practiced just about anywhere, anytime. They do not always require a quiet environment, and most do not require equipment.

One of the simplest relaxation techniques is deep breathing. Deep breathing can actually slow body processes, including heart rate. It involves taking slow, full breaths through the nose, holding the breath for two to four seconds, and then exhaling through the mouth. (Deep breathing must be done slowly to avoid hyperventilation.) As you practice deep breathing, you may want to repeat a relaxing phrase or just the word "relax" to yourself. This technique is simple and inconspicuous enough to be done even when you are in the midst of a stressful situation. You can use it to manage stress and pain or simply to calm yourself or give yourself a few moments before reacting to normal everyday frustrations.

Another type of relaxation technique that requires a bit more imagination is called guided imagery. Imagery is like a planned daydream that transports you to a special relaxing place and state of mind. For example, you might take yourself to a pleasant place that you have been before, such as a favorite fishing spot or a cozy cafe. You might also make up an ideal resting spot, such as a cool alcove in a forest, a warm tropical beach, or a tree-shaded garden. If you're having trouble visualizing, you might consider purchasing a relaxation tape, available at most bookstores or through special catalogues. Better yet, you may want to make your own audio tape or video geared especially to what you find most relaxing.

You'll probably find that imagery works best in a comfortable, quiet environment without television, telephones, or other people (although with practice, you may be able to use it in a less secluded environment as well). This allows you to empty your mind of distractions and focus on the thoughts and emotions that accompany the relaxing images you envision. It can be practiced regularly or used when you are experiencing pain or stress. Ideally, until you become proficient at eliciting the relaxation response, it is helpful to practice one or two times daily for 10 to 20 minutes.

Another more sophisticated way of learning relaxation is through biofeedback. Biofeedback involves the use of equipment that gives feedback from the body related to the level of relaxation that is achieved. This is a tool that, in the hands of a qualified biofeedback therapist, can successfully teach even some of the most tense people to relax (not all individuals are good or willing candidates, but many people find it quite effective).

Biofeedback is now fairly widely used for a variety of problems, including management of pain, tension, stress, anxiety, and high blood pressure. This therapy may be prescribed by your doctor, and in many cases, insurance reimbursement is available. Look for a certified biofeedback therapist. Ask your doctor or other member of your health-care team for a referral or check the yellow pages under "biofeedback."

There are also many other types of relaxation strategies in addition to the ones discussed here. Check your local bookstore for books and workbooks on different methods, or call your local hospital to find out if any classes or workshops are available on relaxation techniques.

FYI

If you are considering the biofeedback option, it is important to remember that the equipment and sensors that are attached to the body do not do anything to you. The equipment merely monitors your body temperature or level of muscle tension. These measures help you to keep track of your body's response as you attempt to relax.

---

12 MASSAGE AWAY PAIN.

You might think of massage therapy as pampering, but it is actually one of the oldest forms of pain management. (Way back in 460 B.C., Hippocrates recommended the process of rubbing the skin and sore joints!) It is now widely used in the management of pain, stress, sports injuries, and traumatic injury to the muscles and joints.

Massage can be performed by a registered massage therapist, a physical therapist, or a willing partner; you can also practice self-massage. In some areas, you may be able to find classes or workshops designed to teach the art of performing therapeutic massage at home. You may even want to check with your health insurer to see if massage therapy is covered, especially if your physician has prescribed massage therapy as part of your arthritis treatment plan.

The following are some basic self-massage techniques; if you have a willing partner, these instructions can also be used to guide your partner in giving you a massage. We've provided instructions for massaging the hands, feet, neck, and shoulders—common targets of arthritis pain. These techniques can be used on other areas as well, such as the arms, abdomen, legs, and even hips. And a gentle face massage can help relieve headache and calm anxiety.

Massage can be performed while you are seated or in a prone position; being comfortable is key. Do not perform massage on a swollen, hot joint that is in a flare, and avoid areas that have skin eruptions, infections, or open wounds. In addition, massage should not be performed on an extremity with known phlebitis (inflammation of a vein) or thrombophlebitis (blood clots in the legs).

SHOULDERS/NECK

1. Using a cupped hand, stroke the side of your neck and your shoulder with the opposite hand. Start at the base of the head and stroke down the side of the neck, across the shoulder, and down the upper arm to the elbow and forearm. Repeat three to four times, then do the same for the opposite shoulder. If you prefer, you can use your fingers to knead the muscles or use deep, small, circular strokes along the same path.

2. Put both hands on the back of your neck, and use the fingertips to knead along the sides of the spine (never directly on the spine). Begin at the base of the neck, and work up into the hairline (see top right).

3. Form a loose fist and gently pound the shoulders. This can help loosen muscles. However, if you find it uncomfortable, skip it.

HANDS

1. Squeeze each finger all along the length of the finger, starting nearest the palm. Then apply gentle pressure along each joint and hold for a few seconds. Hold the end of each finger, gently pull outward, and hold that position (see bottom right).

2. With the thumb of one hand, knead the top and palm of the opposite hand, using small, circular strokes. Then grasp the wrist, gently rotate it, and knead the skin.

3. Gently stroke the area between each finger. Repeat this stroking motion several times. Finish by stroking the hand from the ends of the fingers to the wrist. Repeat until tenseness is released.

FEET

1. Sit upright and rest one foot on the opposite thigh. If your arthritis will not allow you to sit in this position, try lying on your back with both knees bent and, keeping one foot on the floor, pull the other foot toward your chest and rest it on the opposite thigh. Support the foot with one hand; with the other hand, gently massage the toes, one by one, using the same techniques used for the fingers (see number 1 under Hands).

2. Use your knuckles to apply pressure to the sole of the foot. Roll the knuckles back and forth across the bottom of the foot. You can also move the knuckles in a circular motion.

3. Place your thumbs, one atop the other, on the sole. Apply a line of pressure down the center of the sole. Do the same on each side of the sole.

4. Using your fingers, grasp one toe at a time and gently rotate it.

5. Finish your foot massage by rubbing on a lightweight lotion.

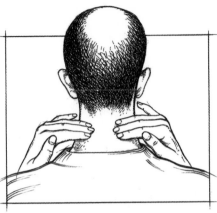

Use your fingertips to gently knead the neck muscles next to your spine. Never massage directly over the spine.

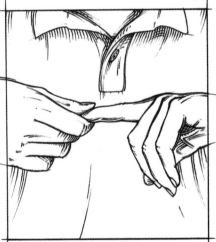

Grasp the end of each finger, gently pull outward, and hold that position for a few seconds.

13 | RESPECT YOUR PAIN.

In this chapter, we've given you several techniques for easing arthritis pain at home. Remember, however, that pain is usually the best indicator that you are placing too much stress on your joints. As such, you need to respect that pain and, in addition to using pain-soothing techniques, make an effort to modify your activities accordingly. The remedies related to joint protection and energy conservation later in the book will help you avoid obstacles that may be increasing your level of pain. You'll also need to pay attention to any increase in your level of pain when you are embarking on an exercise program; being alert to exercise-related pain can help you adjust your level of exertion. Keep in mind, too, that if pain is interfering with your daily activities, you need to tell your doctor.

14 | BE CAREFUL WITH OTC PAIN RELIEVERS.

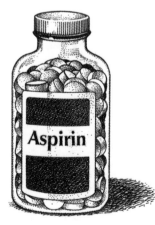

Among the drugs used to treat arthritis pain are over-the-counter (OTC) pain relievers such as aspirin, acetaminophen, ibuprofen, and naproxen. When taken at the dosage recommended on the label, these drugs can be used to relieve occasional, mild arthritis pain, usually without a doctor's supervision. But don't be tempted to exceed the recommended OTC dose without talking to your doctor first. Exceeding the recommended dose may increase the risk and severity of side effects. If you need a stronger dose or need medication on a regular basis, you need to be under your doctor's supervision. What's more, if your pain is moderate to severe, your doctor may decide to prescribe a stronger medication, such as a narcotic analgesic (Darvocet, Tylenol with Codeine, Percodan, Demerol), instead. As with all medications, consult your doctor and/or pharmacist about proper use. And be sure to consult your doctor before taking any other medication, even an over-the-counter drug, in addition to your arthritis medication.

TAKE YOUR MEDICATIONS AS DIRECTED.

In addition to pain medications, there are a variety of drugs used in the treatment of different forms of arthritis. If you have been prescribed a medication for your arthritis, it is vital that you understand the reasons for taking the medication, the possible side effects that you should watch for, and the proper way to take it. You can get this information from your doctor, nurse, or pharmacist. If you don't, you may not get the full benefit of the medication—and you may even do yourself harm.

Consider, for example, the various nonsteroidal anti-inflammatory drugs (NSAIDs) often prescribed to treat arthritis inflammation. NSAIDs include drugs such as aspirin, ibuprofen, naproxen, indomethacin, sulindac, flurbiprofen, meclofenamate, diflunisal, tolmetin, fenoprofen, ketoprofen, and diclofenac. As you may have noticed, some of these, such as aspirin and ibuprofen, were discussed in the previous remedy on pain relievers. It's true that some of these drugs, in low dosages, are used as over-the-counter pain relievers. But to prevent or relieve inflammation, these drugs must be prescribed in much higher dosages. At these higher dosages, however, the risk of side effects is greater, and it becomes essential for a doctor to supervise therapy with these medications. And unlike pain medications, which should be taken only as needed, NSAIDs need to be taken on a regular basis in order to prevent or control inflammation.

Other medications used in the treatment of arthritis include corticosteroids (such as prednisone); disease-modifying anti-rheumatic drugs, sometimes referred to as DMARDs (gold, methotrexate, azathioprine, for example); and specific medications for specific diseases (for example, colchicine, probenecid, and allopurinol for gout). These last medications are not pain relievers, and while they may interfere with the inflammatory process, they do so in a different way than do NSAIDs. They are used only in people with (or with the potential of developing) severe inflammatory disease such as rheumatoid arthritis rather than in those with osteoarthritis. Because of their side effects, they must be taken exactly as directed. For these drugs to be taken safely, your doctor must use frequent laboratory tests to monitor your condition.

Being alert to side effects can make drug therapy safer—and possibly more comfortable—for you. Some side effects, such as chronic diarrhea, may signal a problem and should be reported to your doctor. Other bothersome side effects can often be prevented or eased. For example, stomach upset is a common side effect of NSAIDs and many other types of medication. To help lessen stomach upset from NSAIDs, you can take the medication with food. Other types of arthritis medication, however, should be taken on an empty stomach. To prevent stomach upset with these medications, your doctor may be able to prescribe an additional drug to be taken with the arthritis medication.

Which brings us to a final important aspect of drug therapy: You must understand how and when to take your medications. Some NSAIDs, for example, should be taken once a day; others should be taken two, three, four, or more times daily. Some medications need to be taken daily, others only as needed. Some drugs should be taken with food, others without. With some, you should avoid certain activities while taking the medication. You need to understand and follow as exactly as possible the directions for use. Be sure you ask your doctor or pharmacist for this information if it has not been provided. In addition, ask your doctor how long it takes for the medication to begin working, so you're not tempted to stop taking the medication due to a seeming lack of effect. For some NSAIDs, for example, it may take two to four weeks to determine whether the drug is beneficial for you. If you feel that a medication is no longer effective for you, talk to your doctor before discontinuing it. Also, be sure to ask what you should do if you miss a dose of the drug.

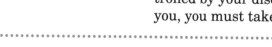

If you find yourself forgetting to take your medication, there are several strategies you can try. You can purchase a divided pill box or wear a watch with an alarm to remind you. You can also try developing a routine for taking your medications. For example, if you're supposed to take the medication once a day on an empty stomach, put the pill bottle next to your alarm clock or your eyeglasses, so you can remember to take the drug first thing in the morning.

Arthritis medications have come a long way. Often, they can mean the difference between maintaining control of your life and being controlled by your disease. But for prescribed medications to be of benefit to you, you must take them responsibly.

CAREFULLY CONSIDER SURGERY.

16

If arthritis pain and decreased function become a burden you can no longer bear, you may need to consider surgery. In rheumatoid arthritis, surgery to replace or repair damaged joints is fairly commonplace. In osteoarthritis, an orthopedic surgeon may recommend surgery if you are so limited in everyday activities or your pain is so severe that it interferes with your quality of life.

Total replacement of the hip, knee, or other affected joints is usually performed by an orthopedic surgeon. Knee and total hip replacements are done fairly routinely; foot- or toe-joint replacements are fairly new. People with severe arthritis of the hands may require reconstruction or replacement of the finger joints.

Depending on your condition, a procedure to repair or realign a joint may be an option. In an osteotomy, for example, bones may be cut and wedged back together to correct orthopedic problems that are the result of arthritis. You may even be a candidate for a less-invasive procedure, such as arthroscopic surgery, in which a small incision is made and damage is repaired using a thin, tubelike surgical instrument.

The decision as to whether surgery is right for you is based on several things. As stated earlier, it is based in part on how much pain and disability you are experiencing. It also depends on which joint is affected; some joints, such as the shoulder, cannot be surgically repaired easily. Your age and physical condition must also be considered.

If surgery has been suggested, discuss the matter in depth with your doctor. Prepare your questions prior to your office visit, and make sure all your questions are answered. Be sure you know why it is being recommended, what it entails, what the risks are, how uncomfortable you can expect to be, how long the recovery period is, and what the chance of improvement is. You'll also need to check into cost and insurance coverage.

If you have severe pain or disability from arthritis, surgery may be the answer. But remember that surgery is serious—and risky—business, and while it may bring relief, it may not cure your condition.

START EXERCISING—BUT GET YOUR DOCTOR'S OK FIRST.

No matter how much your arthritis seems to trip you up, you can take steps to maintain control over your life and your daily activities. One essential step is exercising. Making proper exercise a part of your daily routine helps keep your bones and muscles strong and helps you stay flexible, giving you the physical tools you need to stay in control.

Proper movement of the joints during a carefully planned exercise program helps prevent the loss of calcium from bones, which can make bones brittle and fragile. It helps prevent loss of muscle tone that can make you weak and injury-prone. And it helps nourish cartilage, the tough elastic tissue that covers the ends of bones and helps cushion and protect.

For the person with arthritis, proper exercise is essential. Individuals with chronically painful joints often keep the joints immobile for long periods because they feel better that way. However, if the joints stay immobile or bent for too long, they may become stiff, causing further loss of movement that could eventually lead to deformity.

That doesn't mean you have to—or should—go out and run a marathon. There are varying levels of exercise intensity, and everyone can exercise at one of these levels. Indeed, the most vital type of activity for every person with arthritis is a mild form of exercise called range of motion, or ROM (see remedy 19). ROM exercises involve moving the joints through the full range of movement that the joints allow. You may even be able to do some gentle ROM exercises when your joints are painful or hot (called a "flare"), although you will need to check with your doctor first (some doctors recommend rest during flares). Once the flare has resolved, you should resume a regular exercise routine, including ROM and strengthening exercises, tailored to your abilities (see remedies 19–24).

Before you begin any new exercise program, however, you need to consult your doctor. Your doctor will be able to advise you and your exercise instructor of any limitations you may have. He or she may also refer you to a physical therapist for evaluation.

PLAN AN EXERCISE PROGRAM YOU CAN STICK WITH.

To garner the benefits of exercise, you need to exercise on a regular basis. Sometimes, however, it can be a challenge to stay motivated, especially when you're feeling a bit stiff or fatigued. The following tips can help you plan a program that fits into your daily lifestyle and keeps you interested.

- Remind yourself that exercise is something you can do to help yourself. While improvement may be slow, the results are well worth the effort. If you exercise properly, you can decrease your pain and stiffness, improve your ability to perform everyday tasks, increase your energy level, and even help lessen stress and depression.

- Don't get discouraged if you break your routine. We all have life events and distractions that take us away from even the best laid plans. If you falter from your schedule, just get back to it.

- Choose an activity you like. Exercise should be enjoyable, not torture. If you try one activity and find you don't like it, give another a try. Options include walking (remedy 22), cycling, aquatic exercise (remedy 21), and swimming.

- Blend exercise with socializing. Walk with a friend or in a group so you can encourage and support each other.

- Keep an exercise diary to help you set goals and track progress.

- Start slowly and be realistic about your progress.

- Look for an exercise class designed for individuals with arthritis that focuses on strengthening while avoiding movements that may be harmful to arthritic joints.

- When planning your routine, choose an activity and schedule that you can realistically incorporate into your life. If you enjoy water exercise but have to travel an hour each way to get to the pool, consider whether you'll honestly be willing and able to travel that distance regularly. If not, consider an activity closer to home.

> **FYI**
>
> If you're having trouble developing an exercise plan you can live with, consider consulting a physical therapist or a personal trainer who is knowledgeable about arthritis. These individuals can help you design a program that takes into account your individual physical capabilities, needs, and interests.

19

DO RANGE-OF-MOTION EXERCISES TO DECREASE PAIN AND STIFFNESS.

Many individuals with arthritis experience gel phenomenon, or morning stiffness. It is more common in rheumatoid arthritis but is seen in other forms of arthritis as well. The cause of this symptom is not really known, but it is thought to be related to inactivity, such as during sleep. During prolonged periods of inactivity, fluid is thought to leak out into the tissues, causing swelling and pain. The swelling, in turn, causes stiffness and pain when you attempt to move the affected joint. The swelling and pain usually dissipate during the course of the day, as movement pumps fluid out of the surrounding tissue and into the veins.

There are strategies you can use that may lessen the discomfort associated with morning stiffness. These include using an electric blanket and wearing stretch gloves on your hands at night to keep your joints warm and to help prevent inflammation. Another valuable strategy is to perform range-of-motion (ROM) exercises.

ROM refers to a gentle form of exercise that involves moving the joints back and forth, up and down, from side to side, in every natural direction, as far as they can go. The exercises are aimed at increasing the range of motion of your joints so that you can keep moving and ultimately move more comfortably. They also help to increase your flexibility.

ROM exercises can be done on selected joints prior to getting out of bed. For example, you might put your knee joints through their fullest range possible before getting up and putting weight on them. In addition, you may be able to use ROM exercises to keep up flexibility during a flare (an episode in which the joints are hot and painful), although you will have to discuss this with your doctor first. ROM exercises can also be done before more vigorous exercise, to help warm up your joints, and after exercise, to help you cool down gradually.

Keep in mind, however, that ROM exercises should not replace your regular exercise program. These exercises are not meant to strengthen the muscles that support the joints, nor are they designed to do much for muscle endurance. ROM exercises should be done in conjunction with a program of more vigorous exercise that has been tailored to your specific needs.

When performing ROM exercises, keep these thoughts in mind:

- Begin slowly. Start with five to ten repetitions, if you can, and gradually increase that number.

- Don't push a joint to the point of pain. If you are experiencing pain, you may have extended your range too far.

- Remember to breathe regularly as you do the exercises. Do not hold your breath.

The following are examples of ROM exercises that are commonly recommended for people with arthritis. You may want to put only your affected joints through range of motion, or you may decide to work all joints for increased flexibility.

WRIST AND FINGERS

Always be sure to exercise both hands. You may find it helpful to use a table to support your hands and arms during the exercises.

1. Relax your fingers, and bend your wrist back and forth as far as possible.

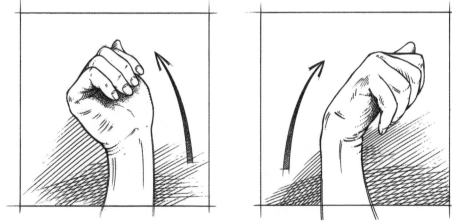

2. Rest your forearm and hand, palm down, flat on a tabletop. Lift each finger as high as it will go. Also lift the thumb. Then, with your fingers together, lift your entire hand while keeping your forearm on the table.

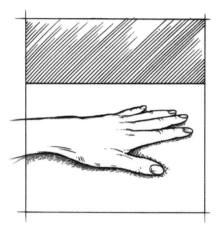 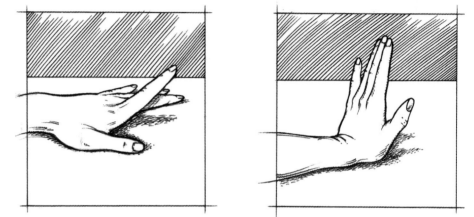

3. Open and close your hand, make a fist, then release.

4. With your hand wide open, touch the tip of each finger to the tip of your thumb. Spread the fingers wide for extended range.

5. Place your hand palm down on a table, with your thumb extended to the side. One by one, slide each finger over to your thumb until all your fingers are together.

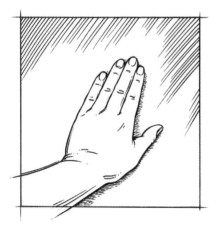 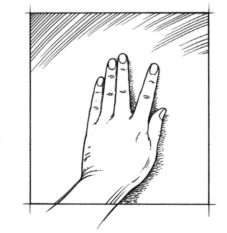 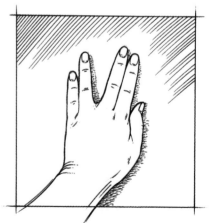

NECK

These exercises can be done while sitting or standing. Remember never to hyperextend the neck directly backward as this puts undue pressure on the cervical spine (upper neck vertebrae).

1. Turn your head slowly and look over your right shoulder, then over your left shoulder.

2. Tilt your head to the left, moving the left ear to the left shoulder; repeat to the right. Don't be alarmed if you hear a cracking sound; it is likely the sound made by the normal movement of bone against bone, known as crepitus.

SHOULDERS

1. Lying on your back, with your arms at your sides, bend your elbows and try to move your upper arms away from your body until they are at right angles to it. Keep your arms on the bed throughout the exercise. (See illustration at right.)

ELBOWS

1. Lying on your back and keeping your upper arms resting on the bed, bend your elbows at right angles so that your forearms are perpendicular to your body. Once in this position, rotate your forearms so that you are alternately looking at the palms and backs of your hands.

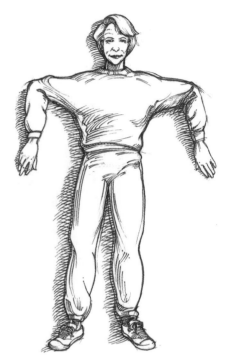

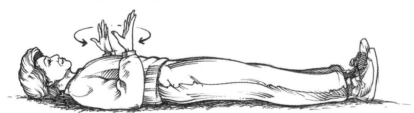

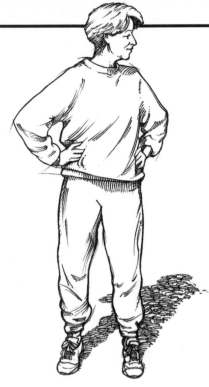

BACK

1. Stand with your hands on your hips and your feet shoulder-width apart. Turn your head and shoulders to the right and then to the left. Keep your hips facing forward throughout. (See illustration at left.)

HIPS

1. Sit on the floor with your legs stretched out in front of you. Roll your legs inward so that your feet point toward each other. Then roll your legs outward so that your feet point away from each other.

KNEES

1. Lie on the floor faceup, with your legs extended. Bring one knee up toward your chest and then back down to the floor. Do four repetitions, then switch legs.

FEET/ANKLES

1. Sit on the floor with your legs extended in front of you. Trace circles in the air with your toes, first clockwise, then counterclockwise. Be sure to rotate your ankles gently. Do several repetitions.

TOES

1. Sit on the floor, with your legs extended in front of you. Flex and extend your toes. If your toes are too stiff, use your hands to gently bend the toes up and down.

INCLUDE STRENGTHENING EXERCISES.

Strong, properly conditioned muscles not only look good, they are essential to supporting and protecting the joints. In particular, strong muscles serve to support the back and spine to help prevent back injuries.

Your regular exercise program will gradually help to strengthen your muscles. However, additional strengthening exercises can be done independent of other forms of active exercise. You may even want to combine your strengthening exercises with your gentle ROM routine.

Usually, strengthening exercises should be done at least once a day but no more than twice daily to avoid fatigue and stress to the muscles and joints. Of course, you need to consider your individual tolerance when determining how often to exercise.

The time of day you select is strictly up to you, but you'll get the best results if you do strengthening exercises when you are not fatigued. This type of exercise may be easier or more comfortable to perform after a warm shower. Some people prefer doing their strengthening exercises before retiring for the evening to promote restful sleep. Whatever time of day you choose, the important point is to do these exercises, as well as your ROM exercises, regularly. They should become as much a part of your daily routine as brushing your teeth.

As you perform your strengthening routine, keep these guidelines in mind:

- Spend a few minutes warming up and stretching to loosen tight muscles and limber up stiff joints before beginning.

- Do your exercises in a logical order beginning with the upper body and progressing to the lower body.

- Perform the movements slowly and smoothly, precisely, and correctly. Distractions such television may cause loss of concentration and improper technique in performing exercises.

- Begin with no more than five repetitions and gradually increase the number of repetitions as your tolerance builds.

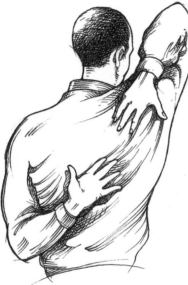

- Change the number of repetitions you do according to the way you feel on any particular day. Listen to your body. If you're having a bad day, don't push yourself.

- Breathe normally. Holding your breath during exercise may cause you to fatigue more rapidly.

The following are examples of strengthening exercises. Keep in mind that a physical therapist who is knowledgeable about the exercise needs and special concerns of people with arthritis can help you establish an individualized strengthening program.

SHOULDERS

1. Raise one arm over your head and reach back with your hand as if you were trying to scratch an itch on your back. Bend the other arm behind your back and reach upward, trying to touch the fingers of the other hand. Repeat using opposite arms. This is a good exercise for both strength and flexibility of the shoulder. (See illustration at left.)

BACK

1. Lie flat on your back on a mat or cushioned floor. (Use a sturdy chair if necessary to lower yourself to the floor.) Pull one knee to your chest and hold for ten seconds; then extend that leg and repeat the movement with the opposite leg. This will stretch the back and prepare it for the following strengthening exercise.

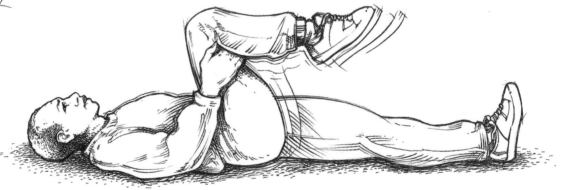

2. Lie on your stomach. Keeping your forearms on the floor, lift your head and shoulders off the floor, placing the weight on your fore-arms. Hold for ten seconds, then release and repeat.

ABDOMINALS

1. Lie on your back with your knees bent and your feet flat on the floor. Slowly raise your head and shoulders off the floor, hold for ten seconds, then release. Be sure to keep your lower back on the floor throughout the exercise. Support your neck with one hand if you have arthritis in the neck region.

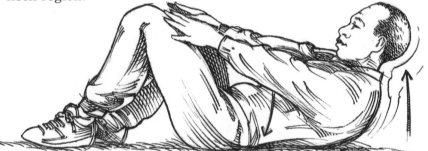

REMINDER

Begin every exercise routine with a warm-up of gentle movement and stretching exercises to prepare the muscles for work. At the end of every workout, cool down for five minutes by decreasing the intensity of your efforts and doing some additional stretching; this will help your body to gradually relax, allow your heart rate to gradually return to normal, and help minimize stiffness.

KNEES

1. While sitting in a firm, sturdy, hard-backed chair, straighten your leg by tightening the thigh muscles. Point your toes straight out in front of you, then up toward the ceiling, working up gradually to ten repetitions, then relax and repeat. Do the same with the other leg.

ANKLES

1. Remain seated in the chair, and raise both feet slightly off the ground. Rotate your ankles to the right and then to the left.

Work toward gradually strengthening all the large muscle groups.

21 TRY AQUATIC EXERCISE.

Aquatics, or water exercise, has long been accepted as an exercise of choice for people with arthritis. Therapeutic water workouts feature a series of specially designed exercises that promote joint flexibility, muscle strength, and relaxation. The buoyancy the water provides allows joints to move through their full range of motion with less stress. Those who have difficulty walking for exercise usually can aquacize, because there's less stress on the back, hips, knees, and feet in the water. For most classes, you don't need to know how to swim (check before you sign up). Here are some tips for selecting and participating in a water exercise class:

- Look for a class sanctioned by the Arthritis Foundation, which has developed a program taught in many locations across the country. To be sanctioned, the instructor must have completed special training. If

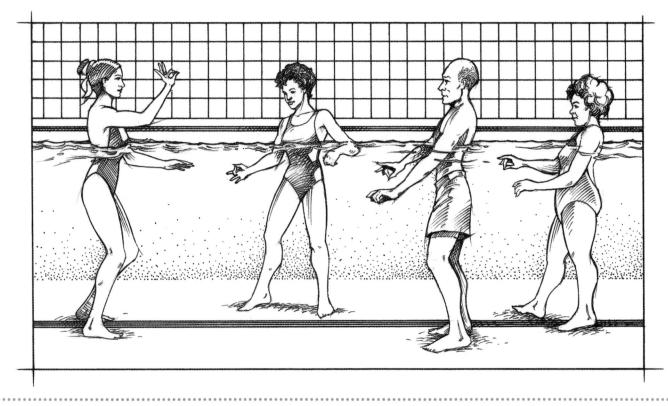

you can't find a sanctioned class, be sure the class you're considering is taught by a qualified instructor who either is a physical or occupational therapist or has some form of certification in water exercise.

- Get your doctor's approval before participating.

- Look for a pool that maintains a water temperature of 84 degrees Fahrenheit (pools for lap swimmers are usually in the 80 to 83 degree range), since you may find cooler water uncomfortable.

- If getting into and out of a pool is tough for you, look for a "therapeutic" pool. Some fitness centers feature pools with ramps or steps with railings leading into the pool and water at only midchest level to promote balance.

- Protect your feet. Regular aquacizing can be irritating to the soles of the feet. Protective nonslip rubber-soled shoes are available at sporting goods stores in a variety of price ranges. These specially designed shoes protect the feet and provide traction in and around the pool.

- If you use a cane or walker in the pool area, make sure rubber-tipped ends are functional and intact to prevent slippage.

- If you wear a swimsuit coverup, make sure it's not touching the floor, so it doesn't trip you up.

- If you want to use the whirlpool at the fitness center, do so only after your water exercise class. The very warm water of the whirlpool may induce fatigue and increase heart rate, potentially depleting your physical resources for exercise.

22 WALK YOURSELF INTO SHAPE.

America is walking! That's right, walking is now the single most popular adult exercise in the United States. And why not? Walking is a form of exercise that is inexpensive (FREE), doesn't require a special skill, and can be done almost any time and any place. It's safe, it's easy, and it makes us look and feel great. And for those who don't feel comfortable walking outdoors, many malls now have extended hours to accommodate walkers.

For people with arthritis, walking is usually an acceptable form of exercise because it strengthens the heart and muscles without putting undue stress on the joints. However, walking may not be for you if you have ankle, foot, knee, or hip problems. If this is the case, consult your doctor or a physical therapist before attempting a walking program.

If you decide you'd like to experience the benefits of a walking program, you'll need to make a commitment to walk regularly—at least three times a week. The only exercise equipment you'll need is a good pair of shoes. Jogging shoes, rather than walking shoes, are recommended for people with arthritis because of the added cushioning they provide.

If you'll be walking outdoors, you'll need to choose your terrain carefully. Uneven ground, loose gravel, potholes, and generally poor walking surfaces can be unsafe. Try to choose a surface that is level and relatively smooth to avoid falls.

Before any walking workout, you'll need to warm up your muscles and joints, especially those of the legs and hips, by walking slowly and doing some gentle stretching. Then walk as briskly as you can, but don't push yourself too hard. Use the "talk test" to keep yourself in a healthy range of exertion: Your breathing should quicken, but you should not be so breathless that you can't carry on a conversation as you walk. Of course, if you experience any pain as you walk, slow down or stop. And if you find that you are sore for two hours or more after a workout, go easier the next time.

CHOOSE WISE WORKOUT WEAR.

Your workout will be more pleasant if you are dressed for the occasion. Choose comfortable clothes that you can get into and out of without assistance, especially if you have difficulty dressing and will be exercising at a health club. Most clubs don't provide assistance with such activities. If you have decreased function in your hands, look for tops that are large enough to get into easily and pants that slide easily over your hips. Try layering clothing, so you can slip off layers as you warm up.

Pay special attention to your shoes. Many forms of arthritis affect the feet, and foot problems are very individual. Select a shoe with a wide toe area that prevents rubbing and pressure. Many shoes are now available with Velcro closures that can be loosened if your feet swell. Look for a shoe with good cushioning and arch support. And try to air out your shoes between workouts, since dampness can lessen a shoe's support.

FOLLOW THE "TWO-HOUR PAIN RULE."

Although exercise plays an important role in the management of arthritis, doing too much can be as bad as doing too little. When you begin your exercise program, you will probably experience some normal discomfort and soreness. You may even be a little more tired than normal at first. However, it's important to recognize the difference between normal soreness and fatigue and overdoing it. How do you do that? Try following the two-hour pain rule: If you have pain or discomfort in your joints for as long as two hours after you've finished your workout, you're probably overdoing it and may need to modify your program. In addition, be careful not to overuse a joint once it begins to feel better, since this can lead to damage.

PLAN AHEAD.

How do you maintain control when you have a disease like arthritis that can flare up unpredictably? How can you commit, weeks ahead of time, to hosting a holiday party or going to a wedding reception when you don't know how bad your arthritis will be or how much energy you'll have? The key is to plan ahead and to be aware of your limits once the event arrives.

Rather than worrying about whether or not you'll be in good enough shape to participate in an expected event, use the time to think about what the activity will entail and what steps you can take ahead of time to make it easier on yourself later. If you'll need to bring a gift, get it and wrap it well in advance. Shop for or select your clothing ahead of time, too. If you're hosting an event, make a list of all that will need to be done, figure out what things can be done ahead of time, and do them gradually and/or delegate some of them. By planning ahead and making some preparations in advance, you'll be able to use the days before the event to get extra rest and conserve your energy.

In addition to preparing for the actual event, you can also prepare—both mentally and physically—for the possibility that your arthritis may flare. Try to be flexible in your thinking. Consider ways that you can still participate even though your arthritis is acting up. Rather than having to miss the event, perhaps you can simply go for a shorter period of time. Perhaps you can reserve special seating ahead of time *in case* your arthritis should flare on that day. Or maybe you can arrange to have a quiet room set aside where you can rest for short periods during the event. Try to have some backup plans in place so that you will not have to miss out on all of the enjoyment because of arthritis discomfort. Keep your thinking and your plans flexible, and you will be able to maintain greater control.

BE ON THE LOOKOUT FOR WAYS TO PREVENT FATIGUE AND CONSERVE ENERGY.

As mentioned previously, most people with arthritis experience fatigue a feeling of extreme tiredness or exhaustion—at least occasionally. The fatigue may result from coping with pain, from depression, or from simply overdoing it. Fatigue may be a side effect of certain arthritis medications. For example, muscle relaxants or tranquilizers that may be part of your treatment can induce drowsiness. And, with certain forms of arthritis, such as lupus or rheumatoid arthritis, the disease process itself may be causing the fatigue.

Fatigue is a symptom that you should pay attention to. Fatigue affects people in different ways, but it usually makes you feel as if you have no energy; you may even feel an overwhelming desire to sleep. Fatigue is also frequently associated with increased sensitivity to pain, a "cranky" attitude, and decreased patience and attention span. As such, it can aggravate your arthritis symptoms, making you more uncomfortable, less alert to possible hazards, and less able to protect your joints.

As discussed in remedy 4, if you are experiencing fatigue, you need to stop and rest. However, you can also take steps in your daily life to *prevent* fatigue from knocking you off your feet in the first place or at least keep it from constantly interfering with your life. The way to do that is to always be alert to ways that you can conserve your energy and sneak rest into your daily routine. The remedies in this section of the book include a variety of specific tactics you can employ in different areas of your life to conserve energy and protect your joints. But you can go beyond these specifics by adjusting your mind-set. Learn to look for ways to make tasks easier or situations more comfortable. Learn to adapt the strategies in this section to other areas and events in your life. The following suggestions may help you start thinking in terms of joint-healthy living:

- Be aware of your surroundings. Pay attention to cues that indicate the environment may be tiring or irritating. For the person with

FYI

Remember to schedule both rest *and* exercise into your daily routine. Rest can help "recharge your batteries;" regular exercise can help increase your endurance overall, so you'll tire less quickly.

arthritis, uncomfortable temperatures, uncomfortable furniture or equipment, constant noise, or stressful conditions affect the levels of fatigue and pain that are experienced. Try to eliminate or modify these conditions, or be prepared to cope with them. If you have a long drive to your workplace, consider keeping the radio turned off and using the silence as a means of relaxing and decreasing outside stimulation. If you frequently find yourself in buildings or rooms that feel chilly to you, learn to keep a sweater with you wherever you go.

- Look for ways to ease strain. If you're waiting for a bus or waiting to enter a theater, turn it into an opportunity to rest by taking a seat on a nearby bench or even leaning against a wall. Be imaginative and creative. One older gentleman who has arthritis did just that during a trip to a flea market with his family. When he started out, he felt fine. About halfway through, however, he began to feel tired. Rather than calling it quits or pushing himself to the point of pain, he improvised. At a nearby booth, he noticed a wooden walking stick for sale. He haggled with the seller over it, bought it for a few dollars, and used it to ease his trip through the flea market.

- Simplify your routines and activities whenever possible. Spending a little extra money on a labor-saving device or taking some time to rearrange your environment and tools can be more than worth it if it allows you to prevent fatigue and pain.

- Try to keep psychological stressors to a minimum; they are a drain on your resources, as well. The benefits of emotional rest have been documented, so a mental health day—or even a few mental health minutes—now and then can truly help boost your energy reserves.

- Decrease your use of caffeine, nicotine, alcohol, and tranquilizers. These all contribute to fatigue when used over time. Also, over-the-counter items like diet pills contain caffeine that may interfere with sleep and mood.

- If fatigue persists despite efforts to combat it, consult your doctor. Anemia or poor nutrition can also cause fatigue.

GET ORGANIZED!

27

Whether your arthritis results in major limitations or minor annoyances, you can benefit from getting organized. Organizing your home, your work, your chores, and your thoughts can help you to do the things you need to do more efficiently, thus helping you conserve energy and prevent fatigue. And by spending less time and energy doing things you need to do, you'll have more to spend resting or doing things you enjoy. Here are some tips to get your life organized:

- **Make lists.** Your friends may call you anal-retentive, but getting into the list-making habit can help you focus and keep you from being overwhelmed. Make a list of things you need to get done each day, each week, each month.

- **Prioritize.** Once you've written down what you need to accomplish, decide which tasks are most important, which can wait another day, and which can be put off until you have more time or energy. Don't expect to do everything on your list; prioritizing can help ensure that you get the most important tasks done.

- **Combine errands.** Check your "To Do" list. Maybe you can get your banking done at the drive-up window on your way to the grocery store. At work, get coffee on your way to the copy machine.

- **Eliminate clutter.** Clutter forces you to go through extra steps—and waste needed energy and time. Visit a store that specializes in home organization, or check the housewares section of your local variety store for containers, shelves, and the like that can help you organize your clutter. And as you sift through that clutter, don't forget to throw out or give away stuff you know you'll never use.

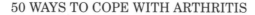

- **Keep supplies together.** Make housework easier by putting your dustcloths, polishes, and cleaners in an apron or lightweight basket you can take from room to room. If your home has more than one bathroom, keep a set of cleaning supplies, toilet paper, soap, and towels in each. When bills arrive, put them in a central location where you also have stamps, envelopes, pens, and checks.

28 USE PROPER POSTURE.

We all know that we should use good posture. We've probably been hearing it since we were kids. But if you have arthritis, using good posture is essential not only for protecting your joints and preventing pain but also for conserving energy.

As odd as it may sound, you can actually waste energy when you are standing in one place or even sitting motionless—if you are using improper posture. Although we may not notice until we fall down, our bodies are constantly working against gravity to keep us in an upright position. The skeleton (especially the spine), the muscles, and the ligaments and tendons share the job of holding us up. With improper alignment, however, the balance is thrown off. Certain areas, such as the bones and joints in the lower back, end up having to support more weight than they were designed to support. To compensate, the muscles have to work harder. Eventually, back strain and even injury may result.

IMPROPER POSTURE

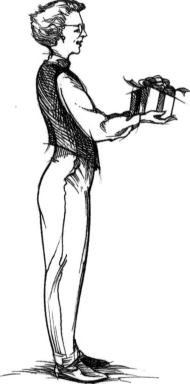

Standing with knees locked and abdominals lax forces your lower back to arch excessively, causing back strain.

The key element of proper posture is maintaining the spine's natural curves. If you looked at your spine from the side, it would look like a somewhat flattened "S." Most often, it's that lower curve of the "S," or the lower back area, that gets abused. We may sit slouched on the couch or over a desk or table, pushing out that lower curve. Or, conversely, we may stand with our knees locked and our shoulders back, exaggerating that lower curve. These postures can stress the muscles and joints of the lower back, cause discomfort, and waste energy.

The following are tips on maintaining proper alignment.

STANDING

- Avoid locking your knees when standing or exercising.

- Pay attention to your pelvis. When you stand with your abdominal muscles lax, the top of the pelvis tends to tilt forward, causing your stomach to bulge forward and your lower back to arch excessively. To prevent this, keep your abdominals tight and your pelvis tucked so that the top of the pelvis faces upward and your tailbone points directly down to the floor.

- Keep your upper body lifted. Imagine a string, attached from the ceiling to the top of your head, lifting your head, neck, and shoulders upward. Keep your shoulders relaxed.

- Alternate standing and sitting whenever possible.

- If you must stand for long periods, place one foot on a low stool, step, or book so it is slightly higher than the other foot; alternate feet occasionally. This will help keep the pelvis properly aligned.

- If you can't keep one foot propped, try shifting your weight from one foot to the other from time to time.

- For long periods of standing, wear shoes with a low, wide heel to provide stability, maintain better alignment, and increase comfort.

SITTING

- If possible, use a chair that supports your lower back and helps maintain the slight curve in your lower spine (see remedy 29).

- If your chair does not provide proper back support, tuck a small pillow or rolled up towel between the chair and your lower back to maintain the lower-back curve. The small inflatable pillows sold for travelers can be handy for this purpose. If you're caught in an unsupportive chair without a pillow or towel, try sliding your forearm behind your back to help support your lower back.

- Sit with your knees slightly higher than your hips and your feet flat on the floor. If necessary, prop your feet on a stool or book to keep your knees at the proper height.

- Change positions frequently if you must sit for long periods. Stand and stretch occasionally, or at least shift your position in the seat.

- When getting out of a chair, keep your back straight. Scoot your buttocks forward toward the edge of the seat. Then use your leg and arm muscles to push yourself up out of the chair. If you push off of the arms of the chair, be sure your hands are facing palm down. Reverse the process to sit back down, bending your knees and using your arms and legs to lower yourself into the chair.

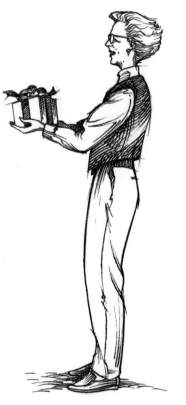

PROPER POSTURE

When standing, keep your knees slightly bent, your abdominals tight, and your pelvis tucked.

29 CHOOSE WISE RESTING PLACES.

To help you maintain proper posture at rest and help ease the strain of getting into and out of a chair or bed, try letting the furniture do some of the work. This can be done either by selecting furniture with specific features or modifying the furniture you already have. Here are some pointers:

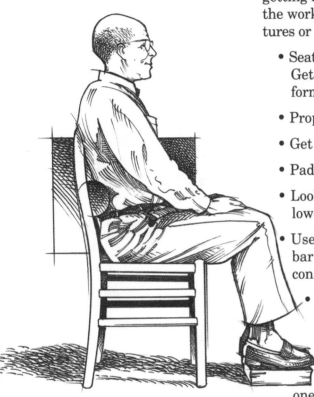

When seated, be sure your lower back is supported and your knees are slightly higher than your hips.

- Seats that are higher than normal will be easier to get into and out of. Get a thick seat cushion or secure your favorite chair to a low platform to increase its height.

- Prop your bed up on blocks to increase its height.

- Get a firm, supportive mattress for your bed.

- Pad hard-bottomed chairs for greater comfort.

- Look for chairs with sturdy armrests that you can use to raise and lower yourself.

- Use chairs with relatively straight backs or ones that provide lumbar support. If your current chairs do not support your lower back, consider purchasing a lumbar-support pillow.

- Consider getting a mechanical chair with a seat that raises you up to a near-standing position at the touch of a button. These tend to be pricey, but depending on your level of disability, you may be able to get some insurance reimbursement.

- If you have stiffness and pain in your neck, try getting at least one chair that has a neck rest or high back.

- Chairs with adjustable footrests can help preserve alignment.

- Place a low, stable stool in the shower to make bathing easier.

- Check sporting goods or camping stores for foldable, portable chairs to bring along to sporting events and other outings.

USE "MOBILITY ENHANCERS" IF NEEDED.

There may be times when your arthritis—or treatments such as surgery—make getting around painful or difficult. Fortunately, there are a variety of "mobility enhancers" available that can help keep you moving and preserve your independence.

- Have railings installed next to your toilet and around your bathtub to make it easier to use these facilities on your own. Be sure all staircases in your home have railings from top to bottom.

- If climbing stairs is difficult for you, look into having a ramp built to your front or back door to facilitate getting into and out of your home.

- If you have trouble getting into and out of chairs, try positioning your favorite chair or sofa next to a halfwall or sturdy piece of furniture that you can grab onto and use to pull yourself up. Or have a railing installed next to your chair or sofa to ease your way (see remedy 29 for more on "helpful" furniture).

- To "unburden" yourself when shopping, doing yard work, or even moving from room to room in your home, try getting a small wagon or cart on wheels so that you can push or pull groceries, supplies, and dishes rather than carrying them. Or try getting a comfortable knapsack or fanny pack to carry items; this will lessen strain to your joints.

- Many larger grocery and department stores offer motorized, sit-in carts for use by shoppers who may have trouble navigating the aisles. Check the stores in your area.

- If you tire easily when walking, consider getting yourself a cane or walking stick.

- If arthritis flares sometimes make walking difficult, talk to your physical therapist about whether a walker or even a wheelchair would be a wise option for you. If you do use one or the other, be sure to get instructions for safe use.

DISTRIBUTE THE LOAD.

One of the most important elements of protecting your joints is learning to distribute the load over larger, stronger joints and larger surface areas. By distributing the weight of objects you are moving or carrying, you reduce stress on weaker joints and help to prevent joint pain. The tips that follow will show you how you can put this principle to work in your everyday activities; for additional instruction in such methods of joint protection, see an occupational therapist.

- When bending over or lifting, always use your leg muscles to lower yourself to avoid stressing the lower back. Bend your knees rather than bending at the waist. If necessary, use a support, such as a sturdy chair or other piece of furniture, to help raise and lower yourself; in this way, you'll be using the muscles in your arms as well to help distribute the load.

- When lifting or carrying objects, hold them close to your body. Objects held closer to the body feel lighter and are less likely to cause you to strain your back.

- Especially if you have hand and finger problems, choose purses, briefcases, and luggage that have shoulder straps. If they don't have shoulder straps, try bending your elbow and looping the straps over your forearm rather than grasping them with your fingers. In addition, pack these items lightly so you don't overstress your shoulder.

- Carry grocery bags in your arms rather than holding the bags by the handles.

- Instead of using your finger to press the nozzle of a spray can or close the lid of a container, put the can or container on a flat surface and use the heel of your hand or your elbow to exert the force.

- When carrying a dish, use a scooping motion with both hands to pick up the dish, and let it rest on your palms rather than pinching it with your fingers. If there's hot food on the plate, use oven mitts that you slip your hands into (rather than potholders that you have to grab with your fingers) to protect your hands.

- Wrap your hands around cups and mugs to pick them up, rather than looping your fingers through the handles. For hot beverages, use an insulated cup to protect your hands from the heat—and keep your beverage warm.

- When wiping a counter or cleaning a window, keep the cloth or sponge flat against the surface and move it around with your open hand instead of grasping it with your fingers.

- When bathing, use a loofah or bathing mitt that you slip your hand into rather than gripping a washcloth in your fingers.

- When pushing open a heavy door, use the side of your forearm rather than just your hand.

- When turning a doorknob, try placing an open hand on each side and, keeping your fingers relaxed, using your palms to twist the knob.

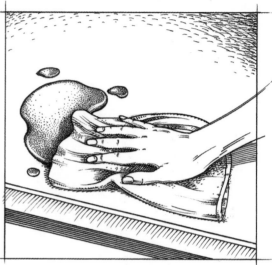

- Use a "hip check" to close drawers.

- Use your palm to turn on wall switches.

- Grasp hanging items, such as dry cleaning, between your two open hands rather than looping your fingers under the hangers.

- Instead of grasping your laundry basket with your fingers, wrap your arms around the basket and carry it close to your chest.

- Rest a book or magazine comfortably on your palms or on a tabletop rather than pinching the edges in your fingers.

- Press down on the pump of a liquid-soap container rather than using your fingers to try and grasp a slippery bar of soap.

32

USE ASSISTIVE DEVICES TO PERFORM EVERYDAY TASKS MORE EASILY.

Assistive equipment or adaptive devices are tools used to simplify activities of daily living. These can vary from simple, inexpensively constructed items to complex custom-designed gadgets. Assistive devices have four basic functions: to compensate for lost function; to alleviate joint stress; to decrease energy demands; and to increase safety. You should not use assistive equipment when you are physically able to complete an activity without excessive joint stress, fatigue, or risk of injury. After all, the demands of daily activities can help you maintain strength and range of motion. Sometimes, you may be able to modify the way you do something (see remedy 31) rather than using supportive equipment. However, there are bound to be times when activities are more difficult for you, and you will need the help of an assistive device.

There are an amazing array of devices available. Some have even hit the mainstream. For example, you are likely to find built-up, padded eating utensils, vegetable peelers, and the like in cooking and housewares stores. Other devices may be a bit harder to find. Check local stores that sell medical supplies and convalescent aids; they may stock some items, be able to order others, or at least have catalogues through which you may be able to order such devices yourself. You can also contact an occupational therapist in your area and ask where assistive devices can be obtained. Another option for some assistive devices is to make your own or modify tools you already have. Here is a sampling of the types of assistive devices available:

FOOD-PREPARATION AND EATING AIDS:

- A special tool for opening sealed cartons, such as cereal boxes

- Jar, bottle, and can openers that are easy on the hands. Some even mount under cabinets.

- A plastic milk-carton holder with a handle to make pouring easier

- Utensils with foam-padding around the handles for easier, more comfortable gripping. You can make these yourself by slipping foam-rubber curlers around the handles of your utensils. Foam-rubber tubing that can be cut to fit is also available. If gripping built-up utensils is still too difficult or painful, you can get utensils that have a hand clip; the clip hooks onto your hand so you don't have to grip the utensil at all.

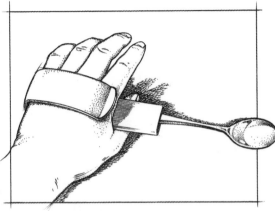

- Built-up kitchen tools such as paring knives, vegetable peelers, and pizza cutters

- A cutting board with a small spike or high edges at one corner to hold food in place and make cutting easier

HYGIENE AIDS:

- Floss holders and threaders

- A toothpaste-tube holder that squeezes the tube for you. You could also buy a brand of toothpaste that comes in a pump dispenser and just use your palm or the edge of your hand to push the pump.

- A nail brush attached to a base that has suction cups on it. You attach the brush to the counter using the suction cups, so you don't have to hold the brush in your fingers. Nail clippers in a similar type of base are also available.

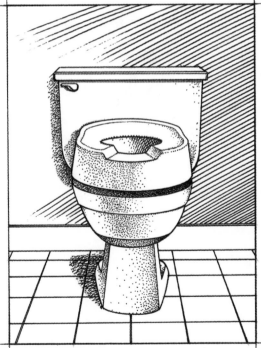

- Built-up grooming aids such as toothbrushes, brushes, and razors, as well as brushes and combs that have long, bendable handles

- An accordion-style holder for your blow dryer that allows hands-free drying. The holder screws into the wall and allows you to adjust the angle and position of the dryer.

- Devices that raise the height of your toilet seat for easier use

DRESSING AIDS:

- Shoe fasteners that slip onto your laces so you don't have to tie them. You could also choose slip-on shoes or shoes with Velcro closures.

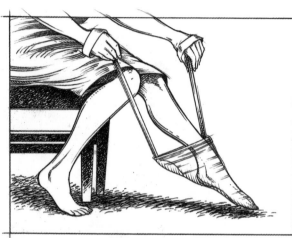

- Shoe- and boot-removing devices that don't require bending over

- Button loops for easier buttoning and unbuttoning

- Dressing aids, such as loops and pinchers with handles of various lengths, that make it easier to put on socks, hose, pants, sweaters, and other clothing

WRITING AND READING AIDS:

- Assorted pencil and pen holders and foam pads to make writing more comfortable

- Special scissors that put less strain on the fingers

- Book holders and page turners

MISCELLANEOUS AIDS:

- An oversized lamp switch that makes it easier to turn the knobs of table and floor lamps

- Playing-card holders and shufflers

- A phone holder with a hand clip that allows you to bring the receiver to your ear without wrapping your fingers around the receiver

- A device that makes it easier to pull an electrical plug out of the socket

- A device for opening car doors that have push-button style handles

GET A HANDLE ON LIFE.

Long handles can be lifesavers—or at least joint savers—for the person with arthritis. Using a long handle on everyday tools can help in three ways. It can help increase leverage, which means you have to exert less force and spend less energy. It can allow you to use a stronger or larger joint to perform a task. And it can help extend your reach, so you don't have to strain or place yourself in a dangerous or uncomfortable position.

To appreciate the benefits of a long handle, consider a faucet with traditional knobs. Turning the knobs applies considerable stress to the fingers and requires a fair amount of strength. If you replace the knobs with long-handled levers (available in home-improvement stores), you increase your leverage and spare your finger joints. If you can't replace your faucet knobs, you can obtain a device that fits over them and creates the same effect; check specialty catalogues or medical-supply stores.

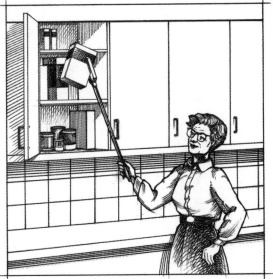

These tips can help you get a better handle on life:

- A device similar to the one that you put on faucet knobs can be used on door knobs. You might even consider replacing your door knobs with handles.

- If turning a key is difficult, attach a homemade handle that allows you to grasp and turn with your whole hand rather than just your fingers. Key holders designed for this purpose are available through specialty catalogues and some medical-supply stores.

- Use a knife to open the flip top of a soda can.

- Use long-handled "pinchers," like those used in stores, to reach light items on high shelves, remove laundry from the dryer, or pick small items off the floor.

- Attach a long handle to a dust pan or sponge to make cleaning easier.

- Use a long-handled shoe horn to put on shoes.

- Slip the hooks of two coat hangers into the loops of your pants and use them to help pull your pants up.

34

SET UP YOUR COOKING AND CLEANING FOR COMFORT.

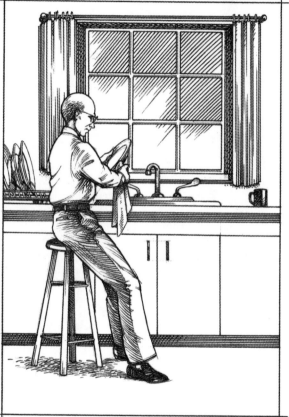

It may sound like a bit of a contradiction to talk of making chores like cooking and cleaning more comfortable. For people with arthritis, however, making these tasks easier on the joints (and on the body as a whole) may be the only way to make them doable.

You can use several basic strategies to make cooking and other household chores...well, less of a chore.

- Adapt the environment to maximize function and conserve energy. In your kitchen, laundry room, or workshop, set up a special place to do certain tasks that use similar equipment. This way, you can keep all the necessary supplies within easy reach. You might even consider duplicating inexpensive items that need to be used in more than one location (get a couple of brooms and dustpans so you can keep one set in the kitchen and one set in the workshop, for example). And if possible, keep a stool or chair near each so that you can sit, or half-sit half-stand, for as many tasks as possible.

To get an idea of what we mean, consider the kitchen. Some of your basic kitchen chores probably include food preparation, cooking/baking, and cleaning up. So try to set up stations for each of these tasks that have all or nearly all of the necessary supplies in them. In your food-preparation station, for example, include various types of knives, cutting boards, mixing bowls, a rolling pin, and other food-prep equipment. In the cooking area, which you should set up by the stove, keep pots, pans, lids, cooking utensils, seasonings, potholders, and the like within easy reach. Consider storing the cooking utensils in easy-access ceramic jugs on the counter nearest the range. In the clean-up center, place your detergent, scrubbers, dish towels, and sponges within arms reach. The more-conveniently placed these items are, the less energy you will waste hunting around for them and moving them back and forth. If you simply don't have the space to keep everything you need in these areas, consider wearing an apron with pockets so you can carry utensils, measuring spoons, and other small items from station to station.

- If possible, store often-used cleaning and cooking supplies on shelves and counters that are between hip and shoulder level. Crouching down to pull supplies out of low shelves or straining to reach high ones can be exhausting and even dangerous. Stock those tougher-to-reach shelves with items that you don't use as often, being sure to put the heavy ones on the low shelves and the light ones above.

- Use labor-saving appliances whenever you can. If possible, invest in a dishwasher, a food processor for chopping and cutting, an electric can opener, a snow and/or leaf blower, a riding mower, or other appliances that will help you conserve energy and give your joints a break. When choosing them, look for joint-friendly features. For portable tools, look for those that are lightweight and easy to handle. When selecting a vacuum, consider getting the type that has all attachments aboard the machine. Be sure it rolls easily on carpets and floors. Look for an on-off switch that can be triggered with your foot, so you don't have to bend over. For other appliances, such as blenders and food processors, look for those with buttons or levers rather than knobs that you have to twist; this way, you can use your palm or the side of your hand, rather than your fingers, to work them.

- If you can't afford certain appliances, look for nonelectric aids. For example, if you can't afford a food processor, ease your chopping chores by getting a manual chopper. This device is basically a cylinder that has a blade attached to a plunger. To chop foods like onions, you simply place the chopper over the onion and, with the palm of your hand, press down several times, depending on the type of cut you need. Also, be sure that kitchen knives and scissors are kept sharp; dull knives force you to grip and press harder and waste energy.

Look for energy-saving cleaning supplies as well. Get a dustpan with a long handle and a mop with a wringer that you can operate without bending over. If you use a duster or blind cleaner, get one with a long handle, or try attaching a lightweight handle to the one you have.

35 PROTECT YOUR JOINTS AT WORK.

Don't forget to check your workplace for ways to conserve energy and protect your joints. The adjustments you can make in this realm, of course, depend on the type of work you do as well as other factors. Some troublesome tasks or situations you may not be able to change, but it's worth the effort to find those that you can. Some of these tips may help:

- If you sit much of the day, get a supportive chair (see remedy 29).

- If your job requires a lot of standing or walking, choose shoes with plenty of cushioning and support and a heel no higher than one inch.

- Whether you sit, stand, or walk all day, use proper posture (see remedy 28).

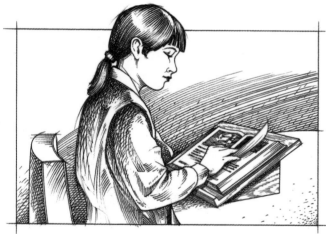

- If possible, adjust the height of your work surface or seat so you're not constantly stooping or bending your joints in stressful positions. If you do a lot of writing or reading, get a portable drafting board or book holder to put on your desk. The board can be set at an angle, so you don't have to hunch over your desk.

- If you spend lots of time on the phone, try a headpiece receiver to lessen stress on your joints.

- Avoid long periods of repetitive movement—whether it's turning bolts on machinery or typing at a computer. See if you can break up tasks that require repetitive movements with those that don't. If your job *is* a repetitive movement, talk to your boss about the possibility of rotating jobs with other workers.

- Organize your work area so that commonly used tools are within easy reach. If you work in more than one area, use an apron, tool belt, or lightweight tote to lug needed items with you.

- Take rest breaks and stretch your muscles at regular intervals. If you stand all day, sit during your break. If you sit for hours, get up and walk—even if it's just to the bathroom.

BATTLE FEAR OF THE DISEASE WITH KNOWLEDGE.

It is very natural to be fearful about a new situation in which you have limited knowledge and feel as if you no longer have control over what is happening to you. Whether it's starting a new job, moving to a new city, or being diagnosed with a disease such as arthritis, fear is a normal reaction. This fear may be even greater for people who have been healthy their entire lives and now find themselves faced with the problem of having to depend on others, including family and medical personnel, to help them perform everyday activities. One step toward fighting the fear and regaining some control is learning as much as you can about your disease.

It's been shown that when people are better educated about their disease, they are more apt to take better care of themselves. Reading this book is a positive step that you have taken to become better educated about your disease. But don't stop here.

One of the best sources of reliable information about your specific condition should be your doctor. Other members of your health-care team are also likely to be valuable resources in this regard. From them, you should be able to get a clear description of what is happening to your body, if and how the disease is likely to progress, and how the various treatment strategies—medications, physical therapy, occupational therapy—may help you to improve.

If you are new to the role of patient, you may find communicating with your health-care providers a bit frustrating at first. It may seem at times that they are speaking a different language, using unfamiliar terms and abbreviations that mean very little to you. It is important, therefore, for you to be assertive and ask for clarification of any terms or statements that you don't understand. Do not be afraid to ask your doctor for an explanation *in English,* not in medical jargon.

If you find it too intimidating to ask your doctor for clarification, it may help to keep in mind that you are a consumer in the health-care arena. There is competition for your business. You have a right to be well in-

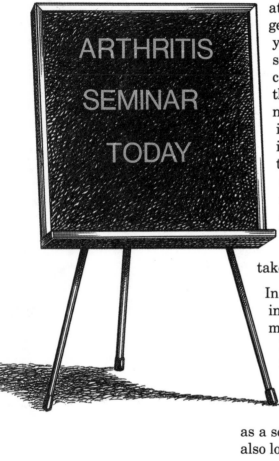

formed, and if your current doctor is unwilling or unable to provide that clarification, you can take your health-care business elsewhere.

If you seem to forget all your questions when you're at the doctor's office, or if you don't come up with questions until after you've left the office, it may help for you to sit down and write out your questions when you're at home. Try as best you can to ask specific questions rather than general ones such as "What's going to happen to me?" When you make your next appointment, tell the nurse or receptionist that you have some questions that you need to discuss with the doctor, so that time can be allotted for this. Then take your list of questions with you to the appointment and check them off as you get them answered. Take notes if you can, since it's easy to forget multiple explanations and instructions when you walk out the office door. You may even find it helpful to bring someone—a friend or relative—with you so that they can listen and take notes for you. Since you are likely to be dealing with a variety of emotions as well as with the sometimes complicated information that your doctor is relaying about your condition, having a support person with you can be truly helpful. Also, be sure to ask your doctor if he or she has any patient-information sheets or brochures about your disease that you can take home with you for reference.

In addition to your health-care team, support groups made up of other individuals who have arthritis can be great sources of practical information and reassurance (see remedy 44). Your local Arthritis Foundation is also a gold mine of information on many aspects of rheumatoid disease (see remedy 45). It has brochures, video programs, and other materials to offer. You can also check local hospitals or local newspaper listings for seminars, workshops, and special programs for people with arthritis. And don't forget the library as a source of useful information. Check not only your public library but also local hospitals to see if they have libraries open to the public.

The information is there if you make the effort to get it. It can be the key to fighting fear and feeling as though you are getting back into the driver's seat.

FIGHT OFF DEPRESSION.

Depression is a normal reaction to stress and tension. It's not surprising, then, that depression is a common side effect of coping with arthritis. The chronic nature of arthritis can bring fears about future functioning. The disease's unpredictability can mean added disappointments in daily life. Coping with pain and physical limitations can force unwanted changes in habits and lifestyle, as well as in self-view. Added to the usual pressures of life, these stressors can trigger depression. Depression can even be a side effect of some arthritis medications.

While depression may be a natural response to stress, it is far from healthy for the person with arthritis. When depressed, the person with arthritis may spend more time focusing on pain and may neglect to keep up with exercises, medications, and other self-care measures. This, in turn, can increase pain and stress, locking the person in a vicious cycle.

That's why it's essential to stay alert to the signs of depression and take steps to keep it from taking hold. The following are some signs to watch for:

- Feelings of sadness, loneliness, or hopelessness
- Neglect of responsibilities and/or personal appearance
- Changes in appetite, weight, and/or sleep patterns
- Poor memory and/or concentration
- Unusual irritability
- Emotional flatness
- Loss of interest in family, friends, and activities that you would normally find enjoyable, such as hobbies, sports, or sex
- Suicidal thoughts or actions
- Physical discomforts including headaches, nausea, and stomach pain

If you begin to notice these signs, take action. Make a concerted effort to keep up with your exercise routine and medication schedule. Force yourself to get out of the house. Make appointments with friends or family for lunch or pleasurable activities. Talk about your feelings with a close friend, family member, or member of the clergy. If these steps don't help, talk to your doctor; he or she can prescribe medication and/or refer you to a qualified therapist.

HINT

If you are feeling depressed, you may find it helpful to talk about your feelings. So if you haven't looked into an arthritis support group before, now may be the time to do so. Simply being around others who have experienced similar fears and frustrations may give you the emotional boost you need. See remedy 44 for more information.

KEEP OPEN LINES OF COMMUNICATION WITH OTHERS— AND WITH YOURSELF.

Often, people who are diagnosed with a chronic illness, such as arthritis, go through stages of adjustment. These stages can carry with them powerful and sometimes confusing emotions—emotions that are confusing not only for the person with the disease but also for those who care about that person. By encouraging yourself through positive self-talk and by talking to your friends and family about how you feel and what you need, you'll have a smoother journey through this adjustment phase.

It may be helpful, first off, to take a look at some of the phases that people typically go through upon being diagnosed with a chronic illness. You may recognize yourself as being in one of them right now.

Perhaps the first emotion experienced is shock—that state of unrealness and numbness. Another common first reaction is disbelief, or denial. When faced with a crisis, there's a natural tendency to want to say "no" to what you are hearing, to think that the doctor must be talking to the wrong patient or that the diagnosis must be wrong. Although it is natural, this stage can be problematic for the person with arthritis because if it lasts too long, it may delay appropriate treatment and self-care.

Once the diagnosis does begin to sink in, you may find yourself angry— angry that you have the disease and angry about what it may mean in terms of your lifestyle and capabilities. Unfortunately, you may find yourself venting some of that anger toward people who care about you and who want to help. This, in turn, may cause feelings of guilt on your part.

Other common feelings include fear (fear of the unknown, fear of how the disease will limit your life, fear that you will become dependent on others) and depression. Remedies 36 and 37 specifically target these two common reactions, but keeping open lines of communication can also help keep fear and depression from standing between you and the support you need.

Although having the support of family and friends during this adjustment period can make the process easier to deal with, you may not always be able to reach out for help. Indeed, the anger, frustration, and disappointment you may feel as a result of your disease may put distance between you and those you care about. But it will be to your benefit if you can let them in on what you're feeling.

For example, if you're feeling angry and frustrated that you can't do as much as you used to because of your arthritis, let your family or friends know that. Sometimes, simply telling someone about it and knowing that someone else knows that you're struggling can help ease your frustration. It can also help them to understand and not take it personally if you are a bit on edge or irritable. They may even be able to help you see and focus on all that you *can* do or on the creative ways you've developed to conserve energy.

Just as important as communicating with people who care about you are the conversations you have with yourself, otherwise known as self-talk. You communicate more with yourself than with anyone else. And you need to be aware of the messages you give yourself and the ways you react to your situation and to other people. For example, being able to admit to yourself that you are feeling bad and telling yourself that it's normal to feel bad sometimes is just as important as conveying those feelings to your partner or friend. It allows you to give yourself a break for being a bit grumpy and may help you catch yourself before you take that grumpiness out on someone you love. Likewise, praising yourself for all that you *do* get accomplished despite your arthritis is much more constructive and self-supportive than dwelling on the limitations that arthritis has caused.

So start talking—and keep talking—to yourself and to the people whom you look to for support. But don't forget that you also need to listen. Those who are close to you must cope with your arthritis too, and they are likely to have questions, fears, and concerns of their own. Good communication is a two-way street. Keep the street open, and together you'll get through the ups and downs of coping with arthritis.

39

BE CREATIVE, FLEXIBLE, AND OPEN ABOUT SEXUAL FRUSTRATIONS.

Discussing the issue of sex and how arthritis might affect it may be uncomfortable for you. It may be uncomfortable for your partner, too. It may even be a topic that your doctor is uncomfortable discussing with you. But it's important not to let discomfort with the subject matter keep you from having a fulfilling sex life despite your arthritis.

Arthritis rarely affects the sexual organs themselves. But that doesn't mean it doesn't affect sexual interactions. Arthritis can have an effect on sexual activity and pleasure in physical and emotional ways. By being

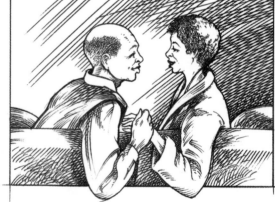

creative and flexible and by being willing to discuss the topic with your partner, however, you are likely to discover that your sex life can be as fulfilling—or perhaps even more fulfilling— than it was before arthritis.

Arthritis pain, fatigue, limited movement, and reduced strength in the hands, arms, or hips can be physical challenges to a fulfilling sex life. Pain is probably one of the greatest barriers, since it is difficult to feel like making love when you are in pain. But there are likely to be ways to keep it from destroying your sex life. For example, taking your analgesic before lovemaking may help reduce the pain.

Creativity in seeking comfortable positions during intercourse can also help reduce or prevent pain and/or make up for weakness or limited movement in certain joints. When there is hip, knee, or back involvement, traditional lovemaking positions may be uncomfortable or impossible. To make lying on your back more comfortable, you might try placing pillows under your knees to relieve back stress. A side-lying position might be more comfortable if one of you has knee problems. For a man with hip problems, having your partner on top may be more comfortable. The point is, don't be afraid to experiment with different positions to find one that is comfortable for both of you.

To help keep fatigue or stiffness from getting in the way of pleasurable sexual activity, try planning ahead for sex. If fatigue is a factor, consider having sex in the morning, when you are more likely to be rested. If you have severe morning stiffness, try the afternoon or evening for sexual activity. Taking a warm bath or shower may also help ease stiffness enough to keep it from interfering with pleasurable sex.

The physical effects of arthritis can also have an emotional impact on sexual relations. A change in appearance or a decrease in mobility or energy level can affect self-image and self-esteem. The person with arthritis may feel less desirable or more fragile. The fear of pain can cause anxiety that makes it difficult for the person to relax and enjoy sex. The partner of the person with arthritis may also be affected emotionally. He or she may worry about causing pain. These emotional effects of arthritis can be conquered by talking openly and honestly. By expressing your fears, you allow your partner the chance to reassure and support you, and you allow yourself to let go of fears that are not warranted. It's important to talk about these issues early on. Otherwise, one partner's fear or discomfort may be taken as rejection by the other partner, causing greater distance and emotional pain. You might even consider discussing these issues with a qualified therapist who has experience with arthritis patients.

Probably the most important aspect of a healthy, pleasurable sex life, however, is the recognition that sexual interaction demands the integration of body, mind, and spirit. Your inner thoughts and your ability to communicate with yourself and your partner have a major influence. A healthy sexual relationship requires trust and compassion. Developing a trusting, loving sexual relationship is challenging for most of us, and for the person with arthritis, it may be more so. Try to take small, slow steps to nurture this process and recognize that sensuality does not always take the form of sex. Having a romantic meal together in a sensual environment, listening to music you both enjoy, bathing or showering together, relaxing in a hot tub, and massaging and caressing each other can all be pleasurable and intimate experiences. Even a gentle touch when your mate is in pain can bring closeness and convey concern and love. Finding ways to overcome the challenges arthritis causes can eventually lead to new self confidence and greater fulfillment for you and your partner both sexually and emotionally.

DON'T FALL FOR QUACKS.

Chronic, incurable diseases like arthritis are prime targets for hucksters, quacks, and well-meaning but misdirected practitioners. The pain, frustration, and disappointments associated with the disease can leave the person with arthritis open to anyone who promises a cure, no matter how bizarre. And there are plenty of people who are playing on that vulnerability. For every dollar spent on legitimate arthritis research, twenty-five dollars is spent on arthritis-related quackery.

Why is such a huge sum of money spent on such methods of treatment? The answer to this question probably has to do with the nature of the symptoms related to arthritis. We have mentioned that pain is the primary reason people with arthritis seek medical treatment, and pain is probably a big reason why people spend money on tonics, herbs, copper bracelets, bee venom, and other unproven treatments. If you experience pain and discomfort for extended periods of time and if medical treatment has not brought sufficient relief, it's not surprising that, out of desperation, you would be tempted to try almost anything.

What's more, because arthritis symptoms often come and go in an unpredictable fashion, it is easy for hucksters to claim that their products or treatments were responsible for relieving or curing arthritis symptoms. They may use testimonials from people whose symptoms seemed to magically disappear when they used the product; in reality, however, the symptoms most likely faded on their own, as they would have done had the person not used the product.

Unproven treatments and "secret" cures are not the answer. Some may be potentially harmful in and of themselves; others may delay or replace proven treatments that *can* be of benefit. Still others simply empty your pocketbook without providing any relief at all. As hard as it may be to hear, there is not yet a proven cure for arthritis.

So how can you protect yourself from unproven and even potentially harmful treatments? Be suspicious if:

- The claims made for a diet or product sound too good to be true. If it sounds too good to be true, it probably is.

- Testimonials rather than scientific studies are used to prove the worth of the diet, product, or treatment. A disease can go into remission or the patient may feel better due to the placebo effect (a beneficial effect that occurs but that cannot be attributed to any special property of the substance).

- You're told that you are one of the "lucky few" to know about this product. Or, it's a "secret" cure that medical professionals don't want to share with the public. Think of it this way: If there were a "secret" cure for arthritis, no doctor or member of a doctor's family would ever suffer from arthritis.

- Accompanying information warns against telling your doctor about using the product.

- The product is sold through a multilevel marketing scheme.

- Phrases like "detoxify your system" or "cleanse your body of numerous poisons" are used.

- The practitioner is clearly profiting from the product. For example, the practitioner insists you buy vitamin supplements from his or her office rather than at your local pharmacy.

If you are tempted by an arthritis "cure" that sounds too good to be true or simply want to know more about a treatment you've heard or read about, consult your doctor or the Arthritis Foundation.

Remember that coping with the emotional aspects of arthritis involves overcoming the frustration, fear, and even desperation that may strike you from time to time. Quack cures are not the answer; they are likely to lead to further disappointment and frustration. Facing the facts and uncertainties of your disease, keeping yourself well-informed, and working to maintain a positive attitude, on the other hand, can help you get through the rough times.

41

EAT HEALTHFULLY.

Eating a healthy, well-balanced diet is important for everyone, but it is especially essential for the person with arthritis. By giving your body enough of the nutrients it needs without too much of those it doesn't, you give it the best chance of functioning well even with arthritis.

The *Dietary Guidelines for Americans,* which were developed by the U.S. Government to improve the nutrient intake of all Americans, are a good place to start on the path to healthier eating. The guidelines recommend that you:

- Eat a variety of foods.

- Maintain a healthy weight.

- Choose a diet low in fat, saturated fat, and cholesterol.

- Choose a diet with plenty of vegetables, fruits, and grain products.

- Use sugars, salt, and alcohol (if you drink at all) only in moderation.

The government not only gave us guidelines, it gave us a new tool to help us make dietary choices that are in keeping with the guidelines and that can help us choose a varied, balanced diet overall. That tool is the Food Guide Pyramid (shown on page 69). The Pyramid represents the recommended daily diet for adults and children over two years of age; it replaces the old "Four Basic Food Groups." As you can see, grains, fruits, and vegetables—the foods that generally provide the most nutritional bang for your buck by supplying a variety of nutrients without an overabundance of fat or calories—make up the greatest portion of the Pyramid. Protein sources take up less room and reflect the fact that most adults get more than enough protein. Within these protein categories, you'd be wise to favor dry beans and peas, low-fat dairy products, and lean meats, fish, and poultry. Fats and sweets, while they add flavor to the diet, should be eaten sparingly.

You'll notice the Pyramid gives a range of servings for each food group. That's because our calorie needs differ. Most women and older adults, as well as people who are less active or are trying to lose weight, will do best with the lowest number of servings from each group. If you choose low-fat and lean foods from these groups and use fats and sweets sparingly, you'll take in about 1,600 calories. Active women, most men, children, and teenage girls should aim for a number in between the lowest and highest number of servings listed. With low-fat choices, this will provide about 2,200 calories. Most active men and teenage boys can eat the maximum number of servings listed to provide about 2,800 calories, assuming low-fat choices.

How much is a serving? The list on the following page will give you an idea.

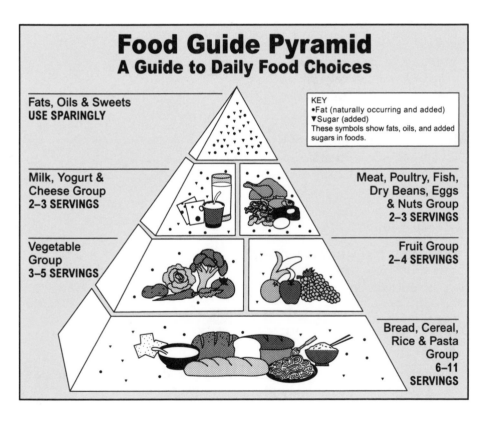

Food Guide Pyramid
A Guide to Daily Food Choices

Fats, Oils & Sweets
USE SPARINGLY

KEY
•Fat (naturally occurring and added)
▼Sugar (added)
These symbols show fats, oils, and added sugars in foods.

Milk, Yogurt & Cheese Group
2–3 SERVINGS

Meat, Poultry, Fish, Dry Beans, Eggs & Nuts Group
2–3 SERVINGS

Vegetable Group
3–5 SERVINGS

Fruit Group
2–4 SERVINGS

Bread, Cereal, Rice & Pasta Group
6–11 SERVINGS

Some examples of single servings in each food group:

Bread, Cereal, Rice & Pasta (Grains) Group

1 slice bread
1 oz. ready-to-eat cereal (see package for cup equivalent)
½ cup cooked cereal, rice, or pasta

Fruit Group

1 medium piece raw fruit (an apple, banana, orange, peach, or plum, for example)
½ cup cut-up raw fruit
½ cup canned fruit
¾ cup fruit juice

Vegetable Group

1 cup raw, leafy vegetables
½ cup cut-up raw vegetables
½ cup cooked vegetables
¾ cup vegetable juice

Meat, Poultry, Fish, Dry Beans, Eggs & Nuts Group

2–3 oz. cooked, lean meat, poultry, or fish
May substitute for 1 oz. meat:
    ½ cup cooked dry beans
    1 egg
    2 tbsp. peanut butter

Milk, Yogurt & Cheese Group

1 cup milk or yogurt
1 ½ oz. natural cheese
2 oz. processed cheese

Fats, Oils & Sweets Group

Use sparingly

By using the *Dietary Guidelines* and the Pyramid, you'll be able to design the kind of diet that your body needs. Be sure to check with your doctor, however, to find out if you have any special dietary needs.

WATCH YOUR WEIGHT.

One of the most important strategies you can use to cope with arthritis is to achieve and maintain a healthy weight. Consider that for every pound of weight you carry over your ideal weight, you place five pounds of added stress on your joints. Weight-bearing joints such as the knees, hips, and spine take the brunt of the strain. In addition, moving that extra weight requires more energy, so you're likely to fatigue more quickly.

Your bathroom scale and mirror may give you some idea of whether you're carrying excess body fat. But talk to your doctor to determine if you are truly overweight and by how much. Together, you can set a goal-weight range. If you have a lot of weight to lose, consult a dietitian to set up a safe, healthy weight-loss plan that suits your needs and tastes.

Whether you go to a dietitian or go it alone, you'll need to:

- Make a long-term commitment to achieving and maintaining a healthy weight. That means viewing the changes you make as a new way of living, not as temporary steps.

- Eschew fad diets and quick-weight-loss plans.

- Follow a low-fat, lower calorie diet. You're more likely to stick with a healthier diet if you make changes gradually.

- Get regular, moderate exercise, such as walking or swimming.

- Set realistic goals. Aim to lose no more than one or two pounds a week on average; faster drops in weight mean you are losing water and possibly muscle in addition to fat. Set short-term (monthly, perhaps) goals that will eventually lead to your goal weight, and reward yourself when you achieve them. See a show, go to a ball game, or buy yourself a small gift. Do not use food as a reward.

- Learn from setbacks. Examine why a setback occurred, consider options for keeping it from occurring again, and get back on your plan.

GET ENOUGH CALCIUM.

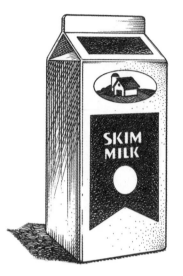

A variety of medications are used to treat rheumatoid disease. Unfortunately, some of these medications, such as prednisone, can cause a loss of calcium from the bones. Over time, this loss of calcium can lead to osteoporosis, in which the bones become porous and brittle. Osteoporosis can lead to fractures, particularly in the hip and spine. Fortunately, you *can* take steps to counter the bone-thinning effects of these drugs. The key is to get plenty of calcium.

The U.S. Recommended Daily Allowance (U.S. RDA) for calcium is 1,000 milligrams per day for women prior to menopause and 1,200 to 1,500 milligrams per day after menopause. For men, the recommendation is 800 milligrams per day. Your doctor or a dietitian can tell you if you'll need to aim at higher levels.

Getting enough calcium in your diet may not be easy. Dairy products are the best source. So if you like and can tolerate dairy products, include several of them in your daily diet. If you don't handle dairy products well, however, you'll need to look harder to find adequate dietary sources. The following table shows some of the better dairy and nondairy sources of calcium.

Food	Calcium (milligrams)	Food	Calcium (milligrams)
Low-fat yogurt, 8 oz.	300–400	Salmon, canned with bones, 3 oz.	181
Milk, skim or whole, 8 oz.	302	Collards, chopped, boiled, ½ cup	179
Cheese, romano, 1 oz.	302	Figs, dried, 5 figs	99
Orange juice, calcium fortified, 8 oz.	300	Kale, boiled, ½ cup	90

If you can't manage to get enough calcium from your diet, you may need to turn to a supplement. You'll need to talk to your doctor about the type of supplement that would be appropriate for you. You might want to ask if one of the antacids made with calcium would be acceptable, since these are inexpensive sources of calcium.

ATTEND A SUPPORT GROUP.

Throughout this book, we've highlighted the need to get accurate information about your disease so you can understand it and be better able to take proper care of yourself. We've also emphasized the need for emotional support to help you cope with arthritis. Support groups can be excellent resources for meeting both those needs.

For the person who has recently been diagnosed with arthritis, a support group can be a vital part of the process of coming to grips with the disease and learning to take steps to control it. Other people with similar problems, concerns, and experiences can help educate and support you during difficult periods. Often, they can provide insights into coping as well as practical tips on managing daily activities.

However, if newly diagnosed, you may be overwhelmed during your first few meetings, because you may not yet be able to absorb all of the realities of having arthritis. Or you may see others with more severe limitations than yourself and be fearful of developing similar problems. If you stay with a group, these fears will usually fade as your knowledge increases.

Choosing a support group that is right for you may take some effort. There are many types of groups, and many styles and approaches. Some groups may be designed for the older adult with arthritis, while others may be geared to the younger adult with rheumatoid arthritis. Some programs are education-oriented, with a variety of informative presentations, and others focus on open discussions about problems or feelings. Try more than one format if you don't feel comfortable in the first group you attend.

Look for a group that is connected to the Arthritis Foundation, a medical facility, or health-care providers. Consider a group with a lay coordinator (someone who has the disease) and a health-care professional who helps facilitate the group. Information about these groups can be found in newspaper listings, through local hospitals, or through your local Arthritis Foundation.

JOIN YOUR LOCAL ARTHRITIS FOUNDATION CHAPTER.

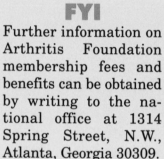

FYI

Further information on Arthritis Foundation membership fees and benefits can be obtained by writing to the national office at 1314 Spring Street, N.W., Atlanta, Georgia 30309.

The slogan of the Arthritis Foundation speaks to the goals of the organization . . . *Your Source for Help and Hope.* The Arthritis Foundation is the only national voluntary health agency seeking the cause, prevention, and cure of the many forms of arthritis. You'd be wise to tap into this valuable resource by joining your local chapter.

Formed in 1948, the Foundation's main purpose is to serve Americans who have arthritis, their families, and the health professionals involved in the care of rheumatoid diseases. The national office, located in Atlanta, facilitates the operations of more than 65 chapters nationwide.

The Foundation's mission includes helping people with arthritis to maintain as high a level of independence as possible. This is promoted through telephone counseling, self-help courses, exercise programs, equipment loans, support groups, and a medication-discount program. The Foundation sponsors programs in public and professional education and helps support individuals studying for careers in rheumatology. The Foundation's work also includes patient advocacy through organized lobbying of legislators on the state and national levels on issues pertinent to arthritis.

Local chapters may vary somewhat in the specific types of programs they offer. However, services generally include: information, referral, counseling, patient education, support groups, exercise programs, fund raising, and support for research in the field of rheumatology. In addition to free literature on a variety of subjects, most chapters offer a physician referral list of rheumatologists in your area, statements on controversial treatments, and information on community resources and volunteer activities.

Your local chapter may have a newsletter that can direct you to programs and community activities and locations of aquatic programs and self-help courses. Membership in the Arthritis Foundation also includes a subscription to the Foundation's national publication, *Arthritis Today.* This monthly information magazine helps keep you current on new treatments, medications, research breakthroughs, and other issues.

GET A SPECIAL PARKING PERMIT.

If your arthritis limits your mobility, consider applying for a handicapped parking permit. Getting such a permit may seem like a big step. You may be concerned about being labeled as "handicapped." But try to consider it as simply another way to conserve your energy and take care of yourself as you cope with arthritis.

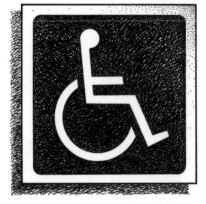

Handicapped parking permits require a signature from your physician. Many doctors keep the necessary form on hand. You can also get one through your state transportation department (check the local telephone directory for the appropriate number to call). You can request a traditional license plate with the universal disabled person logo on it or a laminated window permit that can be moved from vehicle to vehicle and even removed on days when you don't need to use it. The cost of the window permit is usually around $5.

KNOW YOUR RIGHTS.

If arthritis forces you to use a wheelchair or otherwise severely limits you, you need to know your rights under the Americans with Disabilities Act (ADA). In 1990, the ADA was signed into law. Under the ADA, anyone with a physical or mental condition that impairs them must be allowed the same access to establishments and transportation as a person without limitations. The ADA further dictates when such things as ramps and wheelchair-accessible elevators, bathrooms, and buses must be in place. The ADA also specifies that employers may not discriminate against a person with a disability in hiring or promotion if the person is qualified for the job. Write to the state or federal government for detailed information on this powerful tool.

48 PLAN JOINT-FRIENDLY TRAVEL.

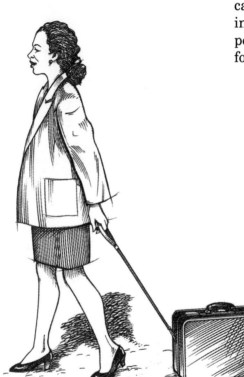

You wouldn't think of taking a trip without packing at least some self-care items. And chances are, you wouldn't go on vacation without making at least some plans to ensure your comfort and enjoyment. For the person with arthritis, such advance planning is essential to a safe, comfortable journey. Here is a "travel bag" of joint-friendly travel tips:

- Find a travel agent willing to discuss your travel needs and preferences, find appropriate accommodations, and keep a list of your needs on file.

- On planes, trains, or buses, request a seat near the front, preferably on the aisle. At the terminal, take advantage of preboarding calls for persons who need extra time in boarding. Reserve a wheelchair or ask to be transported to your gate. Have airline personnel load and unload baggage. Allow ample time between connecting flights.

- Use a carry-on bag with a shoulder strap and luggage on wheels. Consider getting a lightweight, foldable luggage cart.

- Contact motel chains to inquire about ground-floor rooms, elevators, wheelchair ramps, bathroom rails, and other features to increase comfort and save energy. If the motel has a floor plan, ask to have it sent to you ahead of time so you can request a room near facilities you most want or need.

- Get a list of doctors, pharmacies, and health-care services in cities along your travel route, and take your own doctor's phone number with you. Take ample supplies of your medications, copies of your prescriptions, and any regularly used items such as a heating pad, ice pack, pair of stretch gloves, or special pillow.

- If your travels require you to be seated for several hours at a time, get up and stretch your legs or do some range-of-motion exercises in your seat at least once every hour.

- Don't overload your agenda. Schedule time for rest and exercises.

USE SUPPORT SERVICES TO MAINTAIN INDEPENDENCE.

49

In some cases and during certain periods of time, you may require assistance with transportation or support services to help maintain your normal daily activities. There are a variety of resources in place to support you through such rough spots and help you to maintain the highest level of functioning and independence possible.

If driving becomes a problem due to limitations, consult with your local rapid transit or bus services. Many agencies provide vouchers for curb-to-curb transportation for people with physical limitations. Many bus lines also offer reduced fares for people over 65 and those with physical handicaps. Lift-equipped service must also be available on all regular bus routes under the Americans with Disabilities Act. Also, many medical centers now have seniors programs or transportation options offered through their guest relations or patient advocacy departments.

If activities such as dressing or cooking become temporary or long-term problems, home health services such as the Visiting Nurses Association offer nursing care, home health aides, physical or occupational therapy, and other services in the home. There are also a variety of home health agencies, and often their services are reimbursed by Medicare, Medicaid, private health insurance, the Veteran's Administration, or state agencies like United Way.

Other support services include Meals on Wheels for the person who has trouble cooking and is homebound, visitor programs for people who must spend long periods alone, or phone programs to provide support to housebound individuals.

Information about assistance programs can be obtained through state and national health agencies, a social worker, your doctor, or the Arthritis Foundation.

STRIVE FOR WELLNESS.

It may sound like a contradiction to recommend striving for wellness to someone who has a chronic disease such as arthritis. But "wellness" does not refer to being the strongest or most fit or even being free of disease. Wellness refers to a state of being that takes into account limitations and life circumstances. In essence, it refers to being and feeling the best you can under the circumstances—even if those circumstances involve coping with a chronic disease.

No matter what problems your arthritis creates, you can still strive to maintain the highest level of wellness for you as a person. No matter what your state of health, you can try to achieve a positive mental state, acknowledge your limitations, accept that there are some things you simply cannot change, work with those things that you *can* change, and applaud yourself for all that you *are* capable of doing.

Achieving wellness requires that you take charge of yourself and your future rather than simply allowing your disease to dictate how your life will be. It involves educating yourself about arthritis, keeping open lines of communication, and working to adapt and cope with the ups and downs of your disease. Wellness includes discovering your real needs and finding ways to meet them, making choices in the face of uncertainty, respecting the needs of your body, and expressing your needs to others.

In the end, what you need to do to live well with arthritis is not that different from what all people need to do to cope well with the peaks and valleys of life. Granted, arthritis introduces more rough roads and more detours. But it can also teach you to take better care of yourself, to find new ways of viewing and dealing with adversity, and to look forward to and enjoy each and every good day. That's what wellness is all about.